My Twin Flame

JOURNEY OF SEPARATION, SURRENDER, AND RELEASE

Kim,
I hope my story brings some form of healing for you.

In love + His light,
V.C. Pitt

Unconditional Love
Through Spiritual Lessons
and Healing

by *V.C. Pitt*

Copyright © 2022 by V.C. Pitt

All rights reserved. No part of this book may be reproduced or used in any manner without written permission of the copyright owner except for the use of quotations in a book review. For more information, contact: support@mytfjourney.com.

Book Cover courtesy of C. Lyons, artist, and K. Wilcox, photographer
Edited by Michael Ireland, 2022
Proofread by Zora Knauf, 2022
PRESStinely, Author Consulting, Book Marketing & Publishing, 2022

ISBN Paperback #: 979-8-9865366-1-3
ISBN Electronic #: 979-8-9865366-0-6

Library of Congress Control Number: 2022912256

Printed in the United States of America.

V.C. Pitt
United States
www.MyTFJounrey.com

Waiver:
This book is a memoir. The events and experiences detailed within are all true and have been faithfully rendered, as the author remembers them, to the best of her ability. Names and identifying characteristics have been changed, and some events have been compressed, to protect the privacy of the individuals involved, regardless of whether such changes are identified.

Dedication

I want to acknowledge my friends, Melissa, Corrinne, and Beth, who always listened to me during my darkest hours, and supported and loved me through good and bad times. I couldn't have made it through without you.

To my amazing best friend, Samantha. You have been my rock, there with me in the depths of my despair. You have taught me and given me more than I have given to you. Your intuition and advice are always spot on. I am grateful that you are Frick to my Frack. Thanks for the distractions and redirecting me as needed. I love you. You are amazing. Always know that.

Gifted YouTube Spiritual Readers who have given me truth and support along my journey include: Sylvia Escalante (The Enchanted World of Twin Flame), Cristina (Black Rose), Amelia Caddy, Ph.D. (Amelia's Tarot), and Debbie Spachman (Deb Does Readings). You are my beacons of light!

Finally, Erick, you are my Divine Masculine and Twin Flame. You are my other half. My eternal love. Thank you for seeing things in me that I didn't see in myself. You awakened me to start my journey, which triggered me to grow, heal, and work on becoming the best version of myself. Let's get it right in our next lifetime. I will always love you unconditionally. C

Prologue

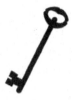

I am from a small town in Tennessee and have an unmistakable southern accent—I'm what some people might call "a country girl." In my childhood and as a teenager, I was naïve and gullible, but was described as sweet and kind. I grew up in a less-than-desirable home with a womanizing, alcoholic, gambling father who abused my mother. Daddy's behavior affected how I felt towards myself. When I stayed with friends, I often wished I had their families instead.

Mama allowed me only a few times to have friends stay over. I didn't understand until I was older how she feared Daddy. My brother, Brian, and I were also scared of him because of his unpredictable anger. She couldn't let me bring classmates home for sleepovers in that dangerous environment. Mama was afraid for her life on more than one occasion. Once, Mama felt something was amiss with her car. She took it to Daddy's father and had him check it. He found that all four of her lug nuts had been loosened.

My earliest memories include Daddy drinking and verbally and physically abusing Mama. She did what she had to do living with him. Once, to protect Brian and me, she pushed us into a closet to shelter us when Daddy's drunken rage resulted in him throwing a kitchen chair across the room.

When I was a small child, her bruises seemed normal to me. That's all I knew. When I asked her as an adult how she stayed married to him, in her own words, she had three choices: kill him, kill herself, or leave. I consider myself fortunate because, after fourteen years of marriage, she left. Mama told me when I was older that the only way Daddy would sign the divorce papers was for her to relinquish custody of us to him. I was ten when the divorce was finalized.

After the divorce, Mama left Tennessee and moved to Mississippi without telling me she was leaving. Daddy told me at the kitchen table on a warm spring day. I hid my emotions—I didn't believe him. *Mama wouldn't leave without telling me.* She did. Although I accepted it, I felt abandoned. This didn't change how much I loved Mama. When I asked, she admitted Daddy didn't want custody; it was a ploy to get out of paying child support. *It was true.* Mama's parents, Granny and Grandpa, became more than grandparents. They were my safety net. Within a year, Brian and I moved to Mississippi, and we lived happily with Mama for the rest of our adolescence. My teen years were happy—well, except for the usual teenage angst.

I was overweight and shy with boys, and had many unrequited crushes. I never dated until the end of my Junior year—after losing weight. Near high school graduation, a friend introduced me to someone whom I saw for three years and later married. I walked down the aisle, knowing I was making a mistake. My self-worth issues caused me to settle for less than I wanted. We were both young and immature, and the marriage ended after eighteen months.

I worked hard but earned little. Living without life's minor comforts, even while married, was normal for me. I thought things would change when I married my second husband, and they did somewhat—but while he was a good person, that marriage didn't last, either. It was a karmic lesson for me.

Although I attended church as a child, traditional religion never resonated with me, and after a few stumbles, I found my way to spirituality, which altered my path and changed my life.

Before my spiritual awakening and second divorce, I recognized that my relationships with Daddy and Brian were making me anxious. When I was upset, I scratched and picked my skin raw. They often used me as a pawn when they were angry at each other. Daddy and Brian were my family, but they weren't good karma within my "soul family"—the reincarnated souls we've shared lives with before. I cut their toxicity out of my life. Years later, I know I made the right decision.

I thought my life would be conventional. I desired to get ahead and worked hard while wearing my heart on my sleeve. I trusted everyone, which set me up for heartache along the way. Over time, Type A tendencies crept in, and I learned self-worth through my job. I pushed myself beyond my limitations. I'm sad to say that I put my job ahead of my family (often). When I met Erick, my Twin Flame, he became my cheerleader. He saw me as a shining star and encouraged me to become a business owner. Over a few years, our business relationship developed into friendship, and then into a combustible affair, followed by unparalleled love and raw heartbreak that pulled me into many dark nights of the soul.

This book is the story of how I faced my childhood core wounds and, through spiritual means, healed and learned to love myself and romantic partners unconditionally. But the road to self-awareness and self-love is sometimes rocky. As you will see, I overcame many trials and tribulations and came through on the other side as an empowered Divine Feminine. I hope reading my story will help you face and heal your own childhood wounds and adult traumas.

I also hope the words in these pages will inspire others who are struggling with their own Twin Flame journey to move forward and heal the wounds that the Twin Flame exposes. I wish you courage on your journey!

All my love,
V.C.

Table Of Contents

Prologue v

Chapter 1 – Awakening 1

Chapter 2 – Sexual Longing 9

Chapter 3 – Emotional Affair 17

Chapter 4 – Consuming, Mirroring Love 31

Chapter 5 – Magnetic Desire 43

Chapter 6 – Separation (The Dark Night of the Soul) 55

Chapter 7 – Connection Through Synchronicity 67

Chapter 8 – Soulmate Recognition 77

Chapter 9 – Death and Acceptance 87

Chapter 10 – Forgiving and Surrendering 101

Chapter 11 – Transforming and Dreaming 109

Chapter 12 – Healing Retreat 119

Chapter 13 – Numbing Out 129

Chapter 14 – Releasing Attachment to Outcome 137

Chapter 15 – Evolving Divine Feminine 145

Epilogue 153

Chapter 1

Awakening

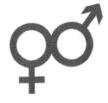

The story I am about to tell you begins when I was in my late forties, living a routine life with my second husband, Greg (now my ex) and our two sons, Kurt and Roman. Kurt was twenty-three, and Roman was seventeen. Greg worked for the State, and I had worked in the healthcare field for over twenty-five years. Kurt was in a technical school, and Roman was nearing high school graduation. We lived a quiet life and were involved with Roman's school. After getting ready in the mornings and seeing Roman off to school, I worked close to nine hours in my multiple offices, rushed home, devoured dinner, and worked again until at least midnight.

Many people would classify me as a workaholic, which is correct, and I have been for over ten years.

At work one day, an unfamiliar feeling came over me. I wanted sex! It was as if a light switch had flipped and I'd become a sixteen-year-old boy. I told Samantha, a colleague, who is also my best friend. We've been friends for forty-five years. She knows me better than anyone. Samantha laughed at me. My sex drive had been non-existent for years. I only had sex when I couldn't put it off any longer.

That afternoon, I received a call from a business coach, Erick, who had supported me when I'd been setting up my business. We had known each other for almost ten years. The first time we met, he came into the office I worked at. I knew he provided business support, and someone suggested I speak with him to prepare for self-employment. After we were introduced, he answered my questions. He was older, but I sensed his sincerity, kindness, and warmth. Something about him felt familiar—it made me think of Daddy—and I wondered if he was an alcoholic.

That evening, I told Greg that I had received some great practical advice to start my business. Later that year, I became a consultant for healthcare offices, and sometimes Erick and I worked in offices simultaneously. Our communications were pleasant. Establishing my role as a consultant, I worked hard, and providers counted on me. As a perfectionist and workaholic, I wanted everything done right and didn't accept less. On many nights, I worked into the early morning hours.

I put pressure on myself to provide results for my clients— they placed their confidence in me. Managers praised my accuracy for billing and accounts receivable and the money I generated for medical offices with which I worked. They sought me out to handle tedious details that would provide financial results and keep small practices from being swallowed by larger entities. Researching rules and earning cash for doctors' offices became second nature to me. I could review and submit medical claims with 99 percent accuracy, which meant offices were paid efficiently and in a timely manner. I was at the top of my career. I was a money generator—which was nice—but I lost bits of me.

My family up-sized to a new home. But even though Greg and I were both earning, it didn't take long for me to become worried about paying our bills. We saved for years to take our kids to Disney World. Greg's work provided flexibility for the kids' schedule, so I worked more and supported us.

Over the next five years, my self-employment expanded. I told Erick I wanted to transition from self-employment to starting a business. He said, "You're going to be a superstar." He presented different options and guided me. My dream of starting my own consulting business became a reality. Another company hired me, and I added more contractors to my business.

The following year, a larger practice hired me. It was the biggest job I had ever taken on, and it changed my life. Due to increased demands in working with four different offices, I was exhausted. No longer happy at a smaller practice I had worked with for a few years, I left. After I quit, someone from that office sent my other offices a scathing email. After reading the email, Erick said, "You're codependent." I didn't understand what that meant, but Erick supported my decision to leave since I'd earn more with the new company.

My business skyrocketed, and Erick was there every step of the way. Greg supported my business, and we faced many professional challenges. His problems trumped mine. He wanted to start a business too, and I supported him. We planned for a year for him to open a business that most people would consider impractical. Unsure of what people might say, I protected Greg's privacy. Erick met us at lunch and felt we had a workable financial plan.

A few months later, Greg quit his job. The brunt of the finances fell to me, and I was determined to earn more. I thought Greg needed free time to transition and start his business. After three months, I became disenchanted—he didn't move forward with his plans; but I said nothing. He worked a few hours in an unrelated job, but there was no incentive for him to work. Greg and I became distant. Anyone looking in from the outside saw nothing but a unified front.

Two years passed. Nothing changed. One weekend, I became weak and nauseous. While taking a shower, I passed out, landed face first on the tiled bathroom floor, and ended up in the emergency room. After several physicians' visits and testing, I learned I had fallen because of a vasovagal response resulting from dehydration.

After this incident, Greg became more supportive. I'd been sleeping on the couch for months because Nikki, our brown Corgi dog, required special care. I felt relieved because I didn't want intimacy anymore. I wanted sex less. It annoyed me that Greg never slept in the living room. After my fall, I slept one night on the bed while Greg slept on the couch, and we alternated the following night. Over the next few months, if he went into the bedroom, I avoided it. Once we went to a work conference together. I attended daytime sessions and worked into the night. He wanted sex. I complied. But after that, he told me we hadn't had sexual relations for seven months. I said, "Really?" I ignored his statement and continued working. Greg and I drifted apart.

I still had a lot of support from Erick. The busier my business got, the more guidance he offered. Over time, Erick saw me become successful. Discussions happened in person and through phone calls. He worked with businesses that needed my skill set, and when he asked, I helped. My gut instincts were almost always right. Our conversations progressed from just business to friendship. General conversation became comfortable.

One day, while Erick and I were in an office talking about business, we were within earshot of two co-workers. I didn't notice them watching us. After Erick left, Sally, the receptionist, said, "I saw you talking to your boyfriend earlier..."

I tried to contain the gasp that escaped my lips and control the scarlet blushing I felt rising in my cheeks. Mortified, I said, "What do you mean by that?"

With a Cheshire grin, "You two always talk," she said.

I sat down in my chair. I didn't like what she was implying.

A couple of years later, Erick called to ask me a business question. I didn't have my laptop with me, so I didn't have an answer. "Samantha and I are headed to a movie," I told him.

"Which movie?" he asked.

I didn't reply.

Unaware he was on speakerphone, Erick said, "Are you going to that *Fifty Shades* movie?"

Samantha grinned.

I felt myself blush. I asked, "What do you want me to say?" I'm sure Erick was laughing—we were so busted! When we hung up, I told Samantha what my co-worker had implied—that Erick was my boyfriend.

"I want to meet him," Samantha said. "I want to see if there is any chemistry."

Samantha is intuitive, and I trust the hits she gets. I took her to Erick's office to introduce the two of them. We had a good rapport, as always. As soon as we left the meeting, I asked, "What do you think?"

"He wants to bend you over his desk and have his way with you," she said. Although I disagreed with her observation, I kept her thoughts in the back of my mind. When it came to my business, my relationship with Erick strengthened. There was a playful tone between us that seemed innocent in my eyes. We became more comfortable with one another. As experts in our respective fields, Erick became a mentor to me.

Paperwork piled up. I needed help. I had to learn an application that gave me anxiety, but Erick was adept with it, which amazed me. He sat next to me and taught me how to enter details correctly. For every error I made, he knew how to correct it. Our hands touched, and I felt the energy between us. That scared me.

We continued exchanging emails that went beyond business. Our work relationship developed undertones of friendship. He saw things in me I didn't see in myself.

Melissa was working with Samantha and me one day. Melissa and I had a twenty-year friendship, and she joined my business as a contractor. She is an amazing co-worker, integral to my business, and we have a special friendship. Samantha and Melissa knew I had a business lunch with Erick at the country club and teased me.

At lunch, Erick was relaxed, but it was all outside my comfort zone. There were women and men in tennis attire, and I felt out of place in casual clothing. We discussed business strategy and reviewed finances. At that point, my heavy workload was stressful, and I pressured myself to work eighteen-hour days. Erick gave me words of encouragement, which reassured me. He surprised me when he ate a fry off my plate. "Did you notice how people are looking at us?" Erick asked, implying that club members were looking at us as if our lunch was not just a business lunch.

With my mind on business, I hadn't noticed. I saw some people look at me as we left the table and walked outside. When I returned to work, Samantha and Melissa asked if anything had happened. I just rolled my eyes at them.

Work never ended. No matter how tired I was, I woke up anywhere from 2:00 a.m. to 5:00 a.m. My mind raced, but sleep eluded me. This lasted for three months, and my anxiety increased. With the marital issues between Greg and me, I resented him. I suggested counseling, and Greg agreed.

We started therapy. "I'm resentful of our family dynamic," I told the counselor. "I work excessive hours and rarely cook. Greg works one day a week. He waits until I get home, and then asks, 'What do you want for dinner?' He prepares some meals, but eating out just seems easier. Can't he make one decision?"

Dissatisfied with my marriage, I talked to Samantha and Mama. I had internalized my truest thoughts of being unhappily married. I could not express frustration to Greg. I became annoyed. He had worked little after quitting his job two years earlier. Samantha didn't understand why I said nothing. I feared conflict (which paralyzed me) and being open with Greg. Why couldn't he have ambition and drive like me? *I was really tired of it.*

During a meeting, Erick and I sat across from each other, closer than I had intended. Because we had a similar sense of humor, I shared details of a recent Vegas work conference trip. "I went to Vegas last month," I told him. "Because I'd mentioned my appreciation for the Magic Mike show, my co-workers suggested to the host that I should be front and center. I was picked to go onstage. I felt like a dirty old woman among the hunky, well-oiled younger men."

Erick laughed.

I told him that THC Edibles are legal in Vegas and I'd overdosed after ingesting a whoopie pie. I ended up being taken by ambulance from a nice restaurant to the emergency room, where they gave me IV fluids. He laughed. I realized I had leaned in. I was feeling comfortable with his leg moving back and forth, close to mine.

Had a similar situation presented itself before, I would have pulled back and crossed no lines. I shy away from interacting with men. I didn't move. Erick began bumping his knee against mine. I met his gaze and didn't look away. He stood up, his body next to my seat, almost inviting me to look at his manhood. But I wouldn't cross that line. Something was different. Nothing physical happened, but I felt the chemistry that I had outright denied. That night, engaging in more than an innocent flirtation entered my mind, although I didn't think sexual thoughts. I imagined him kissing me. My body felt a yearning I had never known before.

Chapter 2
Sexual Longing

Sexual thoughts about Erick set my body ablaze. It was as if there was a gravitational pull towards him. The nights of little sleep transitioned to longing. I confessed to Samantha that I wanted to know how he might kiss. My longing for Erick differed from anything I had known. I couldn't focus because of constant desire and slid down a slippery slope.

I sensed Erick was in an unhappy marriage. A few years earlier, Greg and I had been shopping and had run into Erick and his wife, Karen. She wasn't friendly or engaging. I sensed she wasn't a nice person. She and Erick didn't seem in sync—and she walked away in the middle of the conversation.

I eventually opened up to Erick in an email that I was unhappy in my marriage. I wasn't looking to change anyone's marital status; only to only have a brief sexual encounter. I suggested we meet. I couldn't stop myself. I wanted my senses to come alive. I read my honest thoughts and hit send. *Did I just send that? Oh my God, I did. Holy crap.*

The next morning, I was hesitant and anxious but also excited. *Will Eric call?* It was a busy time of year. But he didn't call. *Oh no... I don't want to lose our professional relationship.* I was anxious. My heart pounded. I hoped I hadn't screwed up. Later, when he called, I was afraid to pick up the phone. But I did. He told me he'd made a colossal business-related error that needed to be rectified with the bank. Our conversation was brief. *Maybe he wasn't thinking... Maybe his mind was on my suggestive email, and that's why he messed up...* I corrected the mistake and texted to let him know. *What now?* I was stumped. *Dammit, why did I send that email?* I struggled with wanting to call him back, but was scared. In a year's time, I had lost twenty-five pounds, but still saw myself as heavy and was not as confident as I wanted to be.

I finished work early the next day and bought a bottle of Fireball whiskey to congratulate Erick's office for getting through another work season. Heart pounding, I walked into his office and chatted with a member of Erick's staff. When Erick rolled his chair from a corner of the room, I couldn't look him in the eye. Erick, his staff, and I opened the Fireball and shared a shot. I drove home, not knowing his thoughts. I felt drawn to him in multiple ways. It went against everything I am.

The following day, Erick called. "Will you have lunch with me?" My mind and body wanted him. We met at a small restaurant by the lake. Erick was in a booth drinking a beer. I sat across from him. He ordered a Jack Daniels, and I ordered my first Mai Tai. I was apprehensive. I couldn't have spoken my thoughts without alcohol, but one thing was certain—I was going to say them.

"What's going on?" Erick asked. I had his full attention.

I reiterated my late-night thoughts. He said nothing.

He's already been unfaithful to his wife.

We talked about many things. He'd planned on taking the afternoon off but had an unexpected project come to the forefront. Three drinks in, I felt bold and seductive as Erick's gaze followed me (and my chest in my low-cut leopard print tank top and short black sweater). With dim lighting, it was difficult to see Erick's eye color, but I saw his pupils were dilated, with little color in the iris. *Is that from drinking or from sexual excitement?* As I stood up, intoxicated in multiple ways, he touched my side to make sure I didn't fall.

As we were by the front entrance, he said, "We can go to my truck and fuck around."

Even with alcohol, I was nervous and said nothing. I walked to my car and turned the air conditioner on, knowing I wouldn't leave until I was sober.

Erick knocked on my passenger window. I rolled the window down. "Let's go back to my truck. I need to get some gas," he said. I believe he wanted me to sober up before driving. I got into his truck and slouched into the passenger seat, removed my sandals, and put my bare feet onto his dash.

"I've always liked country girls," he said. "I'm trying to decide if you could be my partner in crime." *Hmmm. His sidekick.*

We returned to the restaurant for me to get my car, and Erick asked me to follow him to his office and finish work... I had been having Internet issues in my office. I was hesitant, but went.

Back at his office, I was at a workstation outside Erick's office door. He rolled his chair back and looked at me provocatively. We were both distracted. After working for a couple of hours, I left. Erick followed me to a nearby parking lot. He opened my passenger door and leaned in. I tugged at my top, revealing a heavy cleavage, and smiled. *I have never been this forward.* Erick grabbed his crotch, and it turned me on to know he was aroused. He left to meet Karen.

Within thirty minutes, Erick called. The conversation got personal, and I admitted I struggled with orgasm. Erick told me his sexual techniques would help me. The conversation was intoxicating. I clung to every word he said and yearned for him. *Slippery slope... I don't care.*

The following week, Erick invited me to his house to help me with a work project. He understood I couldn't do it alone. I still had time to back out, but I knew I wanted and desired Erick in a way I had never experienced. I wanted to feel him, touch him.

It was a Thursday morning in early May. Erick would be home alone until mid-afternoon. I needed liquid courage to relax me, so I took a small container of peppermint moonshine to Erick's home. We sat beside each other at his dining room table and started working. I noticed his eyes were green. *Like mine.* I opened the glass container of moonshine, and we both drank some. He looked like a kid in the candy store. Erick leaned over to kiss me. "Not yet," I said. "We have work to do."

We reached a stopping point. "Do you want to see the house?" Erick asked. He showed me his bedroom first. I felt he was going to kiss me. It wasn't the best first kiss, but workable. He looked at me, and it felt as if I'd read his mind.

"I am not having sex with you in that bed," I said. *Sex is a given, but it won't be in his marital bed.*

He led me to a barn on his property. "Do you have any pot?" I asked.

He did. After he lit a joint, I inhaled and blew the smoke into his mouth as I exhaled. *I shotgunned him.* It was something I'd never done, but it felt natural between us. We started kissing. I lay back on his couch, and we had gratifying sex. Looking at the surrounding grounds, I felt peaceful. When we were spent, we returned to the house and went back to work, being playful. I sat on his lap in a chair, grinding him. As I left, I told Erick that I've never been with anyone other than Greg since I'd been married. Erick looked at me and said, "Greg is a lucky man." We both broke our marriage vows that afternoon, but I didn't regret it. That night, the day's events echoing in my mind, I slept better.

I felt guilty and scheduled a session with my therapist two mornings later. Aware of my occasional anxiety and depression struggles, and because we were still in family therapy, Greg thought nothing of my appointment. I confessed my infidelity to my therapist. Over the next few days, I experienced a gamut of emotions. I had never cheated on Greg.

Erick called, wanting to meet for lunch. He picked me up at work and we went to a small dive bar. As we talked, he told me stories about his childhood. I learned of his sister's tragic accidental death. He'd been close to her. I could hear the guarded tone in his voice and see the disguised expression on his face when he told me she'd died in a boating accident. Her death had affected his family, and I suspected it was the primary cause of his parents' divorce. He found comfort with his grandmother, just as I did with mine. His mother's name is the same as my grandmother's name. *Coincidental.*

Erick told me a lot about his life that day. He won a sports scholarship to college, but later lost his entitlement because he exchanged harsh words with his coach. His family was financially abundant, but his dad had experienced a reversal of fortune. Erick no longer drove a car, but rode a bicycle on campus. It took him longer to get his college degree than most because Erick repeatedly failed college classes and graduated near the bottom of his class. He couldn't afford his fraternity dues, but because he is likable, he remained part of the fraternity. After he got his degree, he later passed additional testing, which allowed him to become a certified business coach. He had been with many women before he married. He married on the anniversary of his sister's death because he was tired of being sad. They had been married longer than I had and had an older adult son, Ryan. Erick has experienced struggles and challenges, but I admired his perseverance.

After he confessed he wasn't hungry for lunch, Erick said he wanted to take me on the small restaurant table. It was as if everyone else had disappeared. Our gaze connected—I felt a deep longing. I processed his words and remained silent. After we left the restaurant, I asked, "What do you want?"

"Sensuality," he said.

I proposed oral sex. He drove down a quiet road to a small inlet of a lake with a small boat dock. It was quiet, surrounded by some homes in the distance and lots of trees. It was peaceful. No one else was there. I followed through with my offer, and afterward, we returned to work.

We used a project premise to see each other, and I asked him to speak to one office I worked with. As a team, we showcased our business talents. He is smart and articulate, and I admire both traits. He distracted me during the meeting, and I craved melding into the growing familiarity between us.

Continuing as a wife and mom was difficult. I told Mama the reasons I was unhappy in my marriage. Mama asked, "Do you want to be married to Greg for another twenty-five years?"

I replied, "No!" I realized I wanted to leave. I started thinking about leaving my family and divorcing Greg.

At my request, Erick met me and we drove to an isolated park. I told Erick I wanted a divorce, and it wasn't because of him. Erick said, "I wouldn't be able to live with myself if I thought you were ending it because of me. You have a lot of time invested in your marriage. How can you walk away?"

As I was expressing deep thoughts, Erick said, "You are fascinating to watch as you think."

I said, "I'm not happy and I'm choosing to leave."

Erick knew Greg's idea of starting a business and said, "It will put a strain on your marriage." Erick had left home during times of stress, but I never had. I felt closer to him after my confession.

A week later, Greg was oblivious when I carried an overnight bag to my vehicle. I removed him from my business banking account and asked him to meet me in a parking lot. I needed time away. Finding my voice, I blurted out everything I hadn't been able to say. I'd lost respect for him because he hadn't moved forward with his business idea. I wasn't happy in our marriage. Before I left, I said, "Don't call me. I'll call you." I had blindsided him. For the first time in my forty-eight years, I'd focused on myself without regard for anyone or for my responsibilities. I got in my car and drove to meet Erick at a parking lot. I asked him to drop me and my bag off at a car rental facility, and he did. I rented a grey Chevy Camaro. *I was flying the coop.*

In the early afternoon, Erick arrived at the hotel suite I'd rented. Our long afternoon was passionate. He said sex between us was like heaven and the way it's supposed to be. We laughed and enjoyed ourselves. It was everything I wanted, and my body felt satisfaction and pleasure. I had never experienced such intense sex.

Erick returned the following morning. We had sex again that morning, and he was gentle with me. My body and muscles were sore—I could hardly sit down! He left, and I knew I had to end it. When I left the hotel, tears filled my eyes. When I moved forward with what I hoped would be a simple divorce, I didn't want any complications from my involvement with Erick.

Samantha and I went on a road trip. I admitted I had feelings for Erick. She had warned me to not get attached, but I didn't listen. I thought I could handle it and let my guard down. I was tearful over the three days we were together. She listened and supported me. We took a Riverboat Cruise for me to clear my head. I called Greg and said I would come home the following day. I dreaded seeing him.

On our drive home, I texted Erick and told him I wouldn't renew my burner phone, and he called. I said I couldn't see him anymore, but his words persuaded me to continue in what had become a full-blown affair. In less than a month, Erick had become my weakness.

I prepared mentally to see Greg. When I arrived home, we talked more than we had in a few months about our marriage. He was upset. I made no promises—I was exhausted. I am someone who tries to do the right thing, but this time I couldn't.

Chapter 3

Emotional Affair

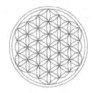

Greg wanted us to attend therapy, and I agreed because I needed time until I figured out how to leave. I had already checked out of our marriage mentally. When I was working, I got a break from marital stress. Continuing therapy alone, I told my therapist I wanted a divorce. At a joint session with Greg, I told him I wanted a divorce. He was devastated. He wanted to work on our marriage.

Erick and I continued seeing each other under the premise of business. We were flying under the radar, and it became more intense. I never thought one person could give me everything I wanted and desired. We discussed *Fifty Shades of Grey*, and Erick mentioned a favorite scene of mine involving a spreader bar. In a vulnerable moment, I asked if he might spank me. The devilish look on his face as I bent over his couch, eagerly awaiting a good spanking... it excited me. I'm not sure what he was thinking, but he delivered some gentle swats to my butt. I said, "Harder, please." He complied. It felt so good. *I can see myself experimenting with BDSM*, I thought.

One hot summer morning, Erick asked me to go with him to the lake. We drove to a secluded wooded area. The sounds of boats on the lake and faint laughter filled the humid air. It felt liberating and free having sex outdoors—and there was a hint of danger in case we were discovered. He pressed me up against a tree and kissed me, then took me on the leaf-covered ground.

We did whatever we wanted, whenever we wanted, and met when our schedules allowed. It became very sordid and erotic. One day, while we were in his office during a heated moment, he thought he heard the door open. Later, he said a couple had come in, overheard us, and left. One Friday afternoon, we were in his office when Karen called. I became very uncomfortable. He sensed my discomfort and walked over to me while talking to her and touched my cheek.

Another morning, Erick and I were in a compromising position when his main office door opened. Partially unclothed, we dressed in record time before the man reached Erick's office. We sat and pretended to be conducting business. I left, relieved that we'd escaped discovery. No matter the chances we took, our passion intensified. He asked me to come to his home on a workday. I arrived and initially, I didn't find him. He was asleep on his couch with a Western playing on TV. I woke him. He wanted me to take a shower with him. When I realized my skirt and his bath rug were wet because the shower door wasn't closed, I told him he should dry the rug so the back didn't mold. I felt guilty when he handed me Karen's hair dryer to use and dry my skirt.

Things became stressful for me at home. I spent afternoons at a local pub and started drinking more. Greg is a smart man and deduced that I was involved with someone. I admitted it but didn't divulge Erick's name to Greg because I imagined how hurt he would be since he knew Erick through my business. Greg even reached out to Erick for a divorce attorney recommendation. Erick didn't return Greg's call. I didn't want to hurt Greg, but it was unavoidable.

After I asked Greg for a divorce, I rented the same hotel and invited Erick again, intending to see him for the last time. I typed a letter to him—I didn't have the courage to tell him face to face that I was ending it. Our affair had started six weeks earlier, and I realized how deep the situation had become. Quiet and reserved, I believe he sensed something was off with me that day.

When Erick came to the hotel, we had good sex. Knowing it would be our last time together, I asked for something special that day. He was more than willing to handcuff me when I asked. I was on my knees, lost my balance, and landed on my shoulder. *Ouch, that hurt.* As he left, I handed him an envelope with business papers and told him there was something important inside. "Read it as soon as you return to the office."

"I will," Erick said.

Inside the envelope was a letter telling him I was ending our affair. I was overcome with sadness. I gathered my belongings and left the hotel. Greg and I met at the bar. I wanted to speak with him about a peaceful resolution of our marriage. As I sat inside, I saw him inside my vehicle. I assumed he had retrieved something. As he walked into the pub, he looked hurt and angry. I was clueless—until he brought a glass growler to my table, with my vibrator inside and the handcuffs on the neck of the bottle. He'd gone through my bag in my vehicle before coming inside. I was mortified. Five people including the bartender saw Greg's outburst before he left, pissed off. I was horrified. Thankfully, the bartender was kind to me.

After Greg had gone, I used my burner phone to text Erick. I was summarizing what had happened and told him I was returning to the hotel for the night. I was unaware of Greg walking in as I texted. "So that's how you did it," he said. *I've been caught.* I looked at him. "I'll never tell you who!" He left, and defeated, I returned to the hotel.

The next morning I called Erick, asking if he'd opened the envelope. "No," he said, "I left it on the desk of a co-worker." *He thought it was just business papers.*

I came unglued. Everything was out of control. "You have to get the letter inside!" My world was spinning. Unsure of how to slow down, I went into self-preservation mode. I avoided home. I had only the clothes I was wearing. A friend let me stay with her for a couple of days. Greg called me, and we talked on the phone. He wanted to meet with me. Greg had been attending church in recent months and wasn't as angry as he could have been. I returned home that evening, and things were quiet. He started asking questions, to which I had to give answers. I made things up. I lied. For the time being, I kept things to myself about Erick's identity.

After reading my letter, Erick didn't want the affair to end. He talked me into continuing, and it took a little convincing. We continued having conversations in person, as well as sending each other texts that grew into heated sexting. Erick asked me to send more than just a few words, which stimulated my creativity and encouraged me to write erotic short stories. It was a genre I excelled at. He knew me well; our minds melded. Our chemistry was unparalleled and went beyond just great sex.

One afternoon, we drove around a winding loop at a local wooded park in mid-afternoon and talked. I said I needed to find a place to live. As I spoke of the future, my thoughts swam. My life was unraveling.

Things became more stressful at home. I stayed on edge. Erick tried to help and guided me to protect myself. Greg continued asking questions. I answered with lies. He thanked me for telling him about my affair. I told Greg I would not see my lover anymore, but I still wanted a divorce. When he asked if it was someone he knew, I lied. I didn't want to hurt him any further. Greg is a good person, but he got comfortable while working minimally and shouldn't have. I thought by giving him information, he could move forward from my infidelity. He had pilfered my belongings at home and took inventory, which is how he knew my vibrator was missing and why he looked in my vehicle at the pub. I felt violated. I shouldn't have been shocked—he is smart.

I needed legal direction and financial protection. I paid an attorney a retainer and explained I wanted everything split 50/50. I meant it. I told Greg I had retained an attorney. I was shocked and angry when he withdrew money from our joint bank account for his own attorney. After that, I took half of the remaining funds and opened another account in my name.

Not knowing what to do, I contacted Erick. He said, "Withdraw what remains."

I said, "I can't. I will get into trouble."

He responded, "No, you won't. You need to."

Although I hesitated, I did what Erick recommended and opened another account, knowing I would split the remaining money after the divorce was final. Later, Greg and I were in the living room. He logged onto the bank website and saw panic on my face. He asked, "What have you done?" I told him I'd withdrawn the money, as I wanted to do things in a fair way, and that after the divorce, I would divide the money. He was furious. He couldn't believe I had done that. Neither could I.

He said his attorney said he could receive eight years of alimony from me. Thank God our youngest son was almost eighteen—he would have tried to get child support.

I stayed away from home in the evenings. To protect my financial interests during divorce proceedings, Erick asked a friend who is an attorney a hypothetical question on my behalf about the affair. The attorney shared information he was given with him.

If I had sex with Greg, he said, it would imply that Greg had forgiven me; that he had accepted the affair. If Greg forgave me, it would cancel out my actions and would be to my benefit. Erick encouraged me to do it, and though I was reluctant, I always followed his recommendations. I tried to tempt Greg under the premise of seeing if there was still chemistry between us. The first time, my advances failed. The following night, I lured and enticed him, and he gave in. But it bothered me.

The following evening, Greg thought we might have a second chance at our marriage. I said, "I didn't want to continue with our marriage."

He said, "You played me!" Things got worse from there. It was the worst advice Erick ever gave me.

On Erick's birthday, we got together early at his place and later, we hung out in the bright sun at the lake. My green eyes are brighter in the sunshine without sunglasses. Green is Erick's favorite color. "You have the prettiest eyes," he said. That surprised me—no one had complimented my eyes before.

At dinner that evening, Greg looked at me and asked, "Did you work hard today?"

I said, "Yes." *Liar.* My intuition alerted me that he knew I was being untruthful. He is intuitive. It felt like a game of cat and mouse.

I proceeded with the divorce and was honest with my attorney about the affair. While at our dining room table, Greg looked at me and only said, "I know," implying he was aware of who my paramour was. I was in denial that he might know it was Erick. He asked, "When have you ever known me to say 'I know' and I don't?" I ignored my gut feeling and shouldn't have, because I thought I'd been careful. I should have listened—he could have followed me. I told Erick, and it made me consider the possibility, although I remained in denial that Greg knew it was Erick.

Greg's life had become very easy since leaving his job with the State. He had worked very little and most mornings, he sat around enjoying coffee while watching political shows on television. *How could he watch me work excessive hours and be content?* Since I was the breadwinner, in addition to Greg being potentially entitled to eight years' alimony, his attorney had said he might get part of my business or a chunk of my financial earnings too. He infuriated me when he said, "Your clothes and shoes could be considered marital property." He threatened to take everything he could from me. I went into fight mode. My business isn't a mom-and-pop shop, but was built on my tenacity, hard work, dedication, and countless nights of little sleep. I thought, *I will be damned if he is getting it.* My attorney wanted to know the order of importance. I said, "He can keep the house, but I don't want to pay alimony, and my business must remain untouched. He can have extra equity in our home if I don't have to name my paramour." I would do whatever was needed to keep Erick from being caught and dragged into my divorce court proceedings.

When I brought up the home equity, Greg said, "You are protecting him. Let me save you a little time." He named four friends my lover might be, but his first thought was Erick. He'd seen my vehicle at Erick's home, and when Erick picked me up from the office. Since he worked one day a week, I believe he had followed and tracked me more than once. At the pub, when he saw me texting on my burner phone, Greg said to me, "You were DEFIANT when you wouldn't tell me who you were having the affair with." My heart jumped into my throat at that moment—my blood pressure was sky high. I texted one word to Erick from my burner phone: "Knows." *Greg had discovered our involvement.*

The following morning, Erick told me he would have to end our business relationship and mail a formal client termination letter to me. I would have to find a new business coach to guide my business.

Upset, I said, "NO!" It seemed unfair. I couldn't bear someone else being my business coach and no longer being in each other's lives. But he had to protect himself. He couldn't be pulled into my divorce, ruin his reputation, and damage his business. People considered him a pillar of the community. I understood, but I would do whatever I needed to do for him to remain in my life. I asked him to meet me at a restaurant and reluctantly, he agreed.

I wore a periwinkle dress that hit every curve.

He asked, "Is anyone looking?"

"No," I said.

He leaned down in the open pizza pub restaurant and kissed me. "You'll have to find another business coach," he said. He gave me two names of other coaches whom he trusted and who would take care of me and my business needs. I felt deep anxiety about him rescinding his business services.

I refused by saying, "No. I don't want anyone else."

"Honey, you have to," he said.

It took little to sway him to continue working with me.

"What color panties are you wearing?" he asked.

"None," I answered. I asked him to go on a beach vacation with me. Although I felt he wanted to, he couldn't. "No," he said.

I left the table first. He met me at my car and we made out.

"Drive to the park," he said. It was the same one we had been to recently.

Although the park wasn't deserted, I found a quiet spot that worked. It had been years since I'd parked and made out in a back seat—it was one of our sexiest times. I straddled him. He squeezed my throat lightly. Instead of being offended, it brought me pleasure. As I looked deeply into his eyes at that moment, it felt as if I was being sucked into his energy. *What is this?!?*

"I will not see you again until you're divorced," he said.

I'll move heaven and earth to complete my divorce.

My attorney required financial paperwork. Erick offered to help, and I met him at his office. "You might lose part of what you have worked for," he said.

I sat on the floor and laid my head on his knee as reality sunk in. I'd hoped he might soothe me, but he didn't even pat my head. *I wonder if he displays emotion towards Karen.*

That afternoon, I worried. *How will I settle financially when the divorce is final?*

Greg and I went to mediation on my forty-ninth birthday. Our settlement was what I had offered, but I also had to make the house payment for two years. After mediation, Greg and I hugged, and I said, "Thank you."

Erick was happy for me. "If Greg was my client," he said, "you wouldn't have come out of it as well." He had served as a witness in court for financial matters in other divorce proceedings.

Erick called late one evening. He'd been drinking and was home alone. He wanted me to come over, but we both knew I couldn't. We talked about spirituality. He explained he could sense others' feelings. I said, "You're empathic, like me."

He said, "Yes."

Since my divorce would be final after the judge signed off, I started thinking more about my upcoming move. I focused on leaving the house I had lived in for ten years. It no longer felt like home. Looking in each room, I only packed what was mine. Greg would keep at least 90 percent of all our possessions. I wanted him and our kids to have almost everything.

During this time, Melissa had told me about a spiritual medium she had seen, who had given her personal information about someone close to her who had died. There was no way the medium could have known the things she shared with Melissa. I began listening to a tarot reader and wanted to learn what she could share with me. When I saw her and described the magnetic connection between Erick and me, she said, "Maybe he is your Twin Flame." She explained it's a spiritual and soul connection, and that we may have experienced past lives together. *Is it possible?* I can find a needle in a haystack...so, I researched Twin Flames. I found so much information. *Holy crap...this could take days to read.*

Twin Flames are people with whom you have a soul connection. They differ from soulmates. Twins are two halves of the same soul who have reincarnated in multiple lifetimes.

They can trigger an uncomfortable emotional response in you—in a way that no one else can—by reflecting your fears or things you don't want to deal with. Twin Flames cause soul growth in one another, and the relationship can be karmic.[1]

Some twins aren't meant to have a romantic relationship. It differs from being with a soulmate—twins challenge the soul. There are multiple stages within this complex situation. It's a magnetic connection that can be tumultuous, especially during the runner/chaser phase. One twin is usually the runner in the relationship; the other is the chaser. If the chaser stops chasing, the runner pursues the chaser—and once the runner ensnares the chaser, then s/he starts running again. And on it goes. Many times twins have a mission to complete here on Earth. *If Erick and I are twins, what is our purpose?* When I had time, I continued researching Twin Flames—there is a lot of information on the Internet! One repeating theme is that Twin Flame relationships wake you up spiritually, whether you like it or not.

There are many symptoms of spiritual awakening, and one of mine includes waking up in the middle of the night with my ears buzzing and not being able to sleep. Ear buzzing differs from tinnitus and is a symptom that the spiritual community refers to as "receiving downloads." I wake up in the middle of the night and receive downloads from the Divine. I had a physician check my ears for any issues, and he found no problems with my hearing. There are times they will muffle for a few seconds, then go back to buzzing. The vibration and pitch can also change. Although I wanted to know more about the symptoms and changes on the Twin Flame spiritual journey, I had to stop researching and focus on my divorce.

---

[1] For more information, including the different stages of the Twin Flame journey, google "Twin Flames."

During the month before our divorce was final, I visited several apartment complexes, looking for a place to live. Erick said it should be nice, which could be costly, but I was looking only to be comfortable. I found a newer, small, modern 782-square-foot apartment that fit my needs and style. After twenty-five years of marriage, I brought only thirty boxes of possessions. My possessions included my furniture and clothing and my challenging pit bull mix, Crystal. As I loaded the truck, Greg cornered me. He couldn't believe I was leaving. I edged my way out, got into the moving truck, and didn't look back. We have never spoken since I left.

I decompressed and settled into my apartment. It was great to be in a relaxing, stress-free environment. The following week, I phoned Erick and asked him to come over. We hadn't seen each other in a month. I grabbed him as soon as he came in. I sensed he missed me, as I did him. We kissed and reconnected, both mentally and physically. We had passionate sex and made up for lost time. I felt joy.

Erick would be alone for a week at home, and I knew we would spend more time together. He came to my apartment. It was nice to be free of being discovered and it was the first full night we'd spent together. We had an Italian dinner. I'm a picky eater and squinted my nose at the suggestion of trying mussels. He backed me up against the kitchen counter and encouraged me to eat one. We were playful, laughing, and happy.

That night, we were free to experiment and had fantasy time. I wore a long, red wig and turquoise dress and became someone different; I went into character and may have scared him a little. He asked, "Where is V.C.?" That made me laugh. I read an erotic story to him in bed, and he listened.

Erick wanted us to get away, to leave the state. We decided on a casino trip two states away. He arrived, and I was apprehensive. Since we had a long drive, I wondered, *What will we talk about? Will he discover he doesn't like me? Are we even going?* I loved Erick and I couldn't contain my emotions. I was going to tell him on our trip. *How will he react?*

Erick is a gentleman, and he carried my bags to his car. I felt uneasy, but we threw caution to the wind and left. Erick knows me, and he sensed I was nervous. I had a playlist ready. He said, "We don't need that," and turned on satellite radio. He sang and sounded good. Erick smiled and said, "Loosen up and sing."

I replied, "I am no American Idol."

He responded, "Everyone can sing."

Finally, I sang and didn't worry. When "Strokin'" by Clarence Carter came on the radio, we grinned at each other. I asked, "Do you know this song?" We belted it out while laughing, talking, and enjoying the rest of the drive with the wind in our hair and the sun's warmth on our faces.

After a few hours, we reached the casino. We checked in under my name, and when the clerk referred to Erick as my husband, I couldn't look him in the eye. I was uncomfortable. Although the casino wasn't full, I wondered, *Will someone recognize us?* We settled into the room and enjoyed each other—no complications. I exhaled. Erick gambled that evening. He was not a winner or loser, but he was at ease in the casino.

In the morning, I slept late. When we went for breakfast, we sat beside each other. When our meals came, Erick had a bite and then fed me with his fork. It was something I have never done, but it felt normal.

As we drove back home, I was quiet. When we arrived, I wasn't sure if he would stay or go. "I need to tell you something. I didn't mean to fall in love with you, but I have." He absorbed it, and I said, "We might be Twin Flames," and I told him why. The look on his face showed I'd thrown him a curve ball. I explained how we felt each other's energy, and that was part of our connection.

Erick revealed he loved me too, and I asked, "Will you make love to me?"

He replied, "It's the same."
No, it's not for me.
We connected, and the sex between us intensified. The pleasure took us to a higher level, and he stayed with me that night.

Erick was attending a football game that afternoon, and I didn't expect to see him. After the game, he called. He wanted to come see me and to go to a nearby movie theater, which was risky, in case anyone saw us.

Later, he told me, "I left the game and walked around town, thinking, 'We weren't supposed to go this far.'" I felt the same way. He didn't elaborate, but intuitively, I felt his mind was spinning after my declaration of love.

We went to a small music venue in town. Erick and I were not discrete in the darkened venue. It had been a special time, even though we knew it was wrong. During a brief break, the singer acknowledged guests in the audience and mentioned "Matt and Diane." Erick said, "There it is." I was puzzled, but the tone of his voice paralyzed me. He and Karen were friends with Matt and Diane and had gone on vacation with them a few years ago.

Holy crap. I felt fear rising in my belly. "What should we do?"

"Nothing, for now," he said. After a few minutes, he said, "Go outside." I turned my head away from the couple, to hide my face, as I walked outside to his car. He walked over and talked to them.

WTF are you doing? I was scared. *What are the odds of something like this happening?* He told me later that Matt looked at him in shock, and Diane wasn't happy. He'd told them I was a relative, but we were sitting close, so I doubted they believed that.

Our free time together was ending, but Erick asked me to come over to his house that evening. We smoked pot, talked about spirituality, and he told me a story about seeing his Guardian Angel. Erick knew he had experienced multiple lifetimes. I loved how we could say anything to each other and we were non-judgmental.

Erick wanted me to stay that night with him.

I should have said no. We were on his marital bed. It was wrong. I never saw myself doing something like that, but he drifted off to sleep with his arm around me. I felt guilty and tried to edge my way out from under his arm. I didn't have the courage to ask, "Will you take me home?" I should have. Every time I moved, he pulled me in closer, and I drifted off to sleep. The next morning, he said, "Lay there and don't move," in a caring way. He had a couple of things to do outside and wanted me to relax, but that would not happen. As I lay in their marital bed, I felt disgusted with myself and waited for him to take me home. I worried a neighbor would see me get into his truck when we left.

Karen was coming home in a couple of days, and it was a waiting game. Erick told me that the woman from the music venue, Diane, had contacted her.

"I downplayed it," he said. I told her, "I was with an extended family member." Our relationship was way past that. Karen told Erick she deserved him being with another woman since she had left him at home, going on a nice vacation without him. It made me wonder about their marriage situation. I waited for the other shoe to drop.

Chapter 4
Consuming, Mirroring Love

Shortly after Karen had arrived home, I attended a work conference and stayed at the hotel where the conference was held. Erick came to the hotel, wanting loving attention. "Things erupted between us," he told me. "I'm a mess. I just need to find a little balance and reassurance."

It had been a hell of a night. "Karen does thousands of dollars' worth of damage to our home once or twice a year." Erick told me. He opened up, and I heard intimate details of a marriage that had been on shaky ground for years. "She hits me," he said. Their argument and noise level upset their dog. His barking woke the neighbors, who texted Erick to see if everything was okay in their home.

She's physically abusive! "You shouldn't have to worry about receiving verbal, emotional, physical, or psychological abuse." *No one should. I'm shocked this is happening.*

Remembering Daddy's anger and abuse, I wanted to show Erick love.

"We argued," Erick told me. "She threatened to call the police... They've been to our home before. Karen hit herself and implied that I'd done it." I shuddered to think of what their home environment might be like given the toxicity between them.

There were marks on his inner forearms. "How did you get those?" I asked. He had taken a screwdriver to himself in case the police were called. *Women can be abusive, too.* His story took me back to my childhood. I remembered Daddy's abuse toward Mama. Hearing how bad things were, I told him, "You are an abused spouse, Erick." He seemed surprised. I wasn't sure how long he'd been a victim. I hurt for him.

"If I move to Montana, would you follow me?" he asked.

"Yes," I replied, without hesitation.

"We would have to move far away, so Karen would leave us alone."

I could see us living together happily.

Erick texted me later and said it was ugly at home. "Know I love you dearly. Thank you for making me feel whole again." He thought he could escape his hell hole.

I texted and said, "I love you and don't forget that." I knew Erick felt the deep love I had for him. I loved him more than I could love anyone. He knew I wanted to be with him, yet he remained at home. It made me question living in a world without us being together. I told him I was selfish and wanted to hold him forever. *We could be happy.* "Don't turn away from us," I said. *How could he remain in a marriage with someone who isn't loving, or in an abusive atmosphere?*

Erick didn't respond for almost three days. When he did, he said, "Your message broke my heart." Things continued between us. "I miss you when we aren't together in the mornings and I dream of you most nights," he told me. "You are beautiful inside and out."

I considered that the ultimate compliment. When he said it, I doubted him and couldn't accept those words. I see myself as an average-looking woman—I stand under five feet, five inches tall and wear a size twelve. I've got a thick middle, big boobs, and a pale complexion. I wear glasses, and my hair can be frizzy at best. I suffer from allergies and I'm a klutz. People tell me that my smile is my best feature. I will always see myself as people saw me when I was younger—as a short, overweight girl whom people thought of as a fat boy. But Erick thought I was beautiful, and that made me love him even more.

One night, Erick worked late and realized he didn't have any alcohol at home. The liquor stores were closed, so he came to my apartment—I had moonshine. I realized he was a functioning alcoholic—he didn't just *want* liquor, he *needed* it. After I told him he was a functioning alcoholic, he responded, "I always show up."

He may "show up," but the truth is I saw he had a real addiction, which concerned me. I loved him no matter his addiction. Erick and I continued picking up on each other's energy. We called it a "mind meld." Energy received in this manner is part of the Twin Flame phenomenon. Our personal, mental, and sexual energy were levels above anything I had ever experienced. When I sensed and felt his energy, it was an unmistakable feeling—like driving fast over a hill and down the other side. He called me his "little Twin Flame."

Besides both of us having green eyes, I see up close with my left eye and far away with the right eye. He mirrors that. We both share some of the same health issues including allergies, sinus issues, and high cholesterol. Twin Flames can share illnesses.

As things became more intimate, Erick and I shared personal details. Men over age fifty sometimes have occasional erectile dysfunction, and he was no exception. His was because of an injury. One morning, he told me how it bothered him when he couldn't maintain an erection, which had never happened before with me. He just wanted to be inside me. I looked into his eyes and hugged him and said, "I don't care. I love you, and it doesn't bother me." But I found a local clinic that specializes in treatment to help what he perceived was a huge issue. He contacted them.

True intimacy grew between us. Erick inspired me and brought me joy. He made sure he satisfied me in multiple ways, and our mental connection was deep. He told me he had only had sex ten times in five years. *I shouldn't be surprised, but I am.*

Mornings with Erick were happy. He brought breakfast, and sometimes I cooked. I'm not a good cook. If I burned something, he would eat it and say he liked it. Our mornings became more frequent as time allowed, and our mind meld increased. One day, Erick wanted to film a video of me as I performed oral sex. "What man doesn't want to be looked at this way?" He told me he had deleted it, but later admitted he still had it—that concerned me.

"Why do you love me?" Erick asked me one day. I wasn't fully vulnerable and couldn't vocalize how I was drawn to his entire essence. He said, "Everyone always wants something from me, but I don't think you do." I wish I could go back and say, "I only want you and your love."

Another time Erick asked me, "Do I know the real you? You're like a kid, childlike and pure. Is this how you really are?"

"Yes."

"There's no one like you," he said.

One morning, I was out of town, 175 miles away. I woke up at 3:00 a.m. I felt Erick's sexual energy. He'd been awake, pleasuring himself, thinking about me and my texts. I felt him intensely.

Before returning home, I visited a psychic medium, and she told me Erick had a big trip planned with Karen in the future. She said he would not change his situation. It was a truth I had to confront. It was killing me to know he wouldn't leave and be with me.

He came over. I didn't ask him about the trip the medium mentioned. Before we got out of bed, I found my courage and asked, "Are you working on your marriage?"

"I am," he said.

I said, "I have to end things. I have to let you go." As I lay with my head on his chest, I told him I had visions of us together. I needed him to go because I was about to cry and felt a large lump forming in my throat.

He said, "You have to get up. You can't stay in bed. We can't depend on others for our own happiness."

It was already painful, and he hadn't even gotten out the door. I hugged him and said goodbye. As soon as the door shut behind him, my tearful explosion hurt my heart. I fell apart. I wailed my grief into my pillow. I balled up on my bed and tried to make it all stop. The floodgate of deep emotions was released, and that evening, I drank heavily. I went within and heard words dropped into my head for the first time, like two people speaking, and I heard, "She's not worth it." It was a channeled message. My self-worth issues made me believe the voice was referring to me, but later a trusted intuitive told me that what I'd heard had referred to his wife.

I told Erick I hoped we could still work together. He agreed and reviewed his horoscope, which said that to live in peace, he needed to restrain his animal impulses and show restraint. He was sorry he hadn't done that with me. Erick said, "He should have known better, and he was an asshole." My head hurt. We wouldn't be together. My tears flowed.

He wasn't an asshole, but quite lovable. It's why I fell for him. I believe he felt guilty about things that had happened in his childhood, all out of his control. He needs to let go of hurt and anger. Erick is in a toxic relationship with a soulmate and karmic partner. Men get abused, but it's not as well-known as other types of domestic abuse. I reiterated that he shouldn't accept any kind of abuse. *How can he accept abusive patterns?*

Through our long text, Erick admitted that they had worked on their marriage for the last twenty years. He didn't want to encourage or mislead me, he said, and I should enjoy my new freedom. Erick said I deserved to be loved and enjoy that love openly. He couldn't give me that. According to him, I am a good, sweet, fine, fun, and sexy-as-hell woman. Erick felt we should take it easy for a bit. I wasn't mad at him, but I was heartbroken.

Erick sent a sexual text. I told him he was an amazing lover, and I loved how he made me feel as a woman. I said the Twin Flame journey was a balance of energy. One person's light is the other's darkness. I elaborated on the visions I'd had of us in different lifetimes together. "I've laid my head on your chest many times before," I said. I didn't want to regret not saying what I needed to, and wasn't trying to make him feel guilty. "I won't forget our time together," I said. "Thank you." Typing those words was difficult. *How can I miss him this much?*

Erick thanked me for an incredible six months and said I was good to him and for him. He wanted me to be happy, not sad. He said I was beautiful, sexy, and that we'd always be more than mere friends. Erick wished we could be together forever, but he couldn't and missed me already. He thought I was a terrific lover, that I awakened part of him, that he loved being with me. He treasured our time together and had no regrets (other than that it had ended). He believed we were Twin Flames. He always felt close to me, like old friends. I tried to comprehend that while he cared for me, he wouldn't leave to be with me.

Erick texted, "Since you cut me loose, I've been obsessed." He was unsure if his quality of life would improve. He'd given up on sex, but I'd made him feel good, wanted, worthwhile, and sexy. Erick hoped he did the same for me.

I was obsessed and didn't want to stop. I was glad he felt that way. I replied, "Never think you aren't." I saw him as a warm, smart, sexy, and a loving person. He may not love me enough to be with me, but I felt loved. "If you decide in the future that you want happiness," I said, "call me. You are incredible."

Erick admitted I had healed him, and he didn't want to stop seeing me. He wanted to make love all night and wanted me to lie on top of him. He wanted to see if it worked out later. I replied that as much as I wanted and craved it, I couldn't continue. Feeling broken inside, I told him I wanted him but couldn't be the third party anymore. He responded that he heard me and agreed. I hoped it meant he was returning, but he didn't write back.

It was hard to keep my mind on work when I was grieving. Every time I thought of Erick, I sobbed. It was uncontrollable grief—I couldn't stop. Because of recent staff changes, I wasn't sure how my business would make it through my distraction. I wasn't sleeping well, and one chilly fall morning, I woke early in darkness to walk Crystal. I didn't have my glasses on, so I couldn't see well, but out of the corner of my eye, I saw a truck idling in front of my neighbor's apartment. I didn't realize until I walked by that it was Erick.

He rolled down his window. "I felt you were awake. I want to talk to you. Can I buy you breakfast?" I was apprehensive, but I agreed. *Why did he come?* I agreed and walked Crystal quickly. He brought me a bacon, egg, and cheese biscuit. I let him into my apartment.

He wanted to return to my life. I'm unsure who missed the other more. He is the one person I couldn't say no to. Before he left, I showed him my Harry Potter scarf and pulled it in front of my chest. He walked over to me, and I stood still as he wrapped the scarf around my face, leaving my nose and lips exposed. My body was aware of him and I waited in anticipation of what he might do. The hair on my arms was standing on end. My senses were heightened. I craved him and whatever he was about to do. When his is lips met mine, it was sweet, yet it was the most erotic kiss I've ever experienced. We began our emotional affair again, although sex wasn't part of it that early morning.

After a few nights, I received a message: "I love you. Please help me. Do you love me?"

Without hesitation, I said, "Yes. What can I do to help you?" We were yin/yang energy. I wanted to be with him in every way, to be close to him. I wanted to be with him all the time.

"I've decided," Erick said. "I'm leaving and need help. What we have is real. There just isn't enough of me. I am tired of being beaten up by her. I don't understand her actions."

"I want to give you happiness."

"Sweetpea," he replied. "I want to grab you in my arms. Help me figure it out. We are fighting again... She is frigging killing me."

I knew their home situation was worse. Erick was tired of their fights and wanted to leave. There would be violence and hell to pay if he left. He told me, "I love you and your beautiful smiling green eyes."

I reassured him. "I will do anything to help you."

He admitted to being a strong person, and said that if he decided to leave, it wouldn't be hard on him. Erick saw and felt things intuitively. His intuition is on point.

The two of us weren't the only ones sinning. He alluded to Karen having a problem living with herself. *That is why she hit him.*

He asked, "Can you live with my alcohol addiction?"

"I would." *Without hesitation.* Daddy was a mean alcoholic. Erick wasn't. I wanted him to have less stress in his life, for him to feel loved, and allow me to be his rock.

Erick asked, "Are we really twins?"

"I believe we are."

"We could keep coming together," he said. "We are having a lot of fun."

Is this just fun for him?! That stung. I was hurt. "You should research Twin Flames on the Internet and decide."

Erick said, "It's become more than fun, but I'm not wired to walk out or leave a life we have spent many years making." He admitted he lived much of his life in a less-than-happy state. Through prayer and making a choice to be happy, he's lived a wonderful life. He asked, "Why do you think I love to hear you giggle and see your genuine happiness?"

Erick loved that about me and our connection. He loved me, but he was "wired" to perform as duty called. Erick admitted it would fuck him up because the longer we were together, the more he felt he had to protect me, and he wanted to be honorable towards me. He wasn't sure where we could go with us. Erick loved and respected me; he didn't like me not having all of him, but he didn't have it in him to make it happen. *WTF?*

I exploded. I thought we would be together. I told him we had to separate. I wouldn't ask him to leave since he was "wired to do the right thing." I refused to stay in limbo. Erick acknowledged that I was right, that we would try it. I was so hurt and asked, "Why did you tell me you were leaving?"

"I was pissed off. Every time I saw you, you were happy to see me."

"You shouldn't have told me you were leaving if you didn't mean it." Also, he knew I could give him everything. In anger, I said, "You could remove yourself from an unhappy, abusive, and manipulative relationship." Erick said he deserved that, but he wanted to see what happened. He wouldn't apologize because he wanted to see me again. I loved him but wouldn't be his second choice. When we stepped away from each other's energy, I felt sad, angry, and hurt. I'm embarrassed to admit it, but all I could do was grab a pillow and scream into it while jumping up and down, stomping around my apartment like a two-year-old child. I wanted to hit something.

Samantha had an engagement party that night. An acquaintance asked me about a serious fall I'd taken in my bathroom the year prior. Looking through my cell phone to find the date, I found a photo of me in the ER and the exact date it happened. I felt the air being sucked from my lungs. It was November 11: 11/11. *1111 is the Twin Flame number!* Although I had seen Angel number sequences for three months when working and on license plates, the date was beyond coincidence. *Synchronicity.* Since I had figured out we had telepathy between us, I sent him energy when I awoke. He texted me later and said, "Darn it, stop. You were sending me energy early today, weren't you?"

I said, "No," and he asked, "Really? It was early." *Busted.*

What did he want me to say? I tried to leave him alone, but I couldn't help myself. He was in my thoughts constantly. He didn't know how to respond. I said, "I could ask you the same. Are you sending me energy?" Erick said he wasn't trying to do that. But he did. We both sent and felt each other's energy. This type of telepathy happens between Twin Flames.

It was supernatural. Some people will doubt it is possible. If I hadn't experienced it myself, sending energy to Erick, and receiving it in return, I wouldn't think it could happen. I have heard of it happening between birth twins, of course. My grandpa was an identical twin, and he and his twin brother shared telepathic experiences. It's an internal radar or frequency that is felt between twins. Erick and I are on the same vibrational frequency. *Our energy is a perfect match, which is why we felt each other's energy so strongly.*

That evening, when I saw his number on caller ID, I almost didn't answer my phone. But I did—he was thirty seconds away from my door. I put my bowl of ice cream away and let him inside my apartment. He wanted to see me. I sat in my chair as he stood beside me so he couldn't tempt me. He touched me and said, "I know my mama loves me, Ryan loves me, and you love me."

Guarded, I only listened.

He told me had never had a connection like ours with anyone before. He hugged my stiffened body. I couldn't speak, knowing he had been with many women before he married. The most touching part was him saying no one had ever opened his heart until me. I knew he loved me.

I should have said, "I can't continue," but again, I let him back into my life.

The telepathy between us continued. Our stolen time together became all either of us wanted. The mutual respect between us, our friendship, and our loving sex was all-consuming and intimate. We shared so much. I felt Erick's guard slip away—he could be himself without fear in my presence. I felt loved on a higher level. It had taken forty-nine years for me to feel love like this. One morning at dawn, while we were in bed, two things happened. As my body lay against his, I felt our hearts beat in unison. *Did that just happen?* He felt it too. Almost immediately, I saw his face morph into a younger version of a man I hadn't seen before. I didn't tell Erick what I had seen—but it was inexplicable. Intuitively, I knew the face I'd seen was from a past life we'd shared.

On another morning, we lay in bed and I was talking about my newfound spirituality. I had visited a spiritual church. It made more sense to me than any religious service I had attended. As my mind wandered and I talked about the 5D world, the metaphysical world beyond the physical plane of existence, I said, "I can see a special place for us. There's a creek rushing through a grassy valley with a large tree to one side of the field. There are white and purple wildflowers in bunches on the soft, grassy field." Erick wanted to add mountains with an overlook to our place. We created that special place in our minds, where we could always go when we wanted or needed to.

The next week, Erick had a business meeting that required him to fly out of town. He stopped by early that morning, looking handsome in a navy sports jacket. He wanted to see me for just ten minutes because he missed me. We sat on the loveseat, and I curled my body around his. Texts sent to me that day included a song message, "You Are So Beautiful to Me." Eloquent words and his intelligence drew me in, and he always let me know he was thinking of me.

I had been seeing Angel numbers more often, and Erick mentioned seeing a number sequence while he was on his business trip. *He was seeing Angel numbers, too.* Angels communicate with us by sending us numbers. There are many repetitive numbers that the Divine sends us. Current sequences I saw were triple and quadruple numbers, everything from 111 to 9999. I'm observant of details that most people overlook. I continued allowing numbers to find me through billboards, license plates, and purchase receipts, then I searched the Internet to find out what each one meant. I remained open to what the Angels wanted to tell me.

Chapter 5
Magnetic Desire

Out of nowhere, an acquaintance threatened my business. Erick walked me through handling a situation that had the potential to cripple what I had worked so hard to build. He reassured and calmed me, as no one else can. Sensing how off-kilter I was, he asked me to come in during business hours for a meeting. (He surprised me when he closed his office door and kissed me—there were other people in the office!) He helped me jump through a major hurdle, and I emerged stronger. Erick had his own work problem not long after mine, and I reassured him. I loved that we supported each other. My words helped him, and we became closer.

One day, we were together in my apartment. Erick was getting dressed and walked into the living room wearing just jeans. As an older man, Erick's chest was defined, and he turned me on. I told him, "I don't know which is my favorite body part." He grinned while flexing his biceps for me. It made him happy that I appreciated his body. He told me he was drawn to me and described me as "every man's dream that's bold enough to play with fire." I'd embraced my sexuality late in my adult life, and I was vulnerable with him. Erick said, "Part of why I am attracted to you is your confidence." He didn't realize that his appreciation of all of me increased my confidence.

One day, I heard Erick on the phone with Karen—he called her "Honey Bun." Later, he called me "Honey Bun." I said, "Don't call me that." After he left, I texted, "If you are going to call me by a pet name, it should be a name other than what you call your wife."

"I'm sorry, Honey Bee," Erick said. I forgave him.

It had been two months since my divorce was final. Thanksgiving was my first major holiday alone. I was in a lonely, vulnerable state. I met another man that weekend, drank a lot on Saturday night, and had a one-night stand. It is something I'm not proud of and had never done before. It was a foreign concept to me.

The next time I saw Erick, he told me, "You are a good person."

I couldn't look him in the eye but said, "No, I'm not." I never admitted that I'd slept with someone else. I told him later that I had met the owner of a recording studio and we'd hung out. There was a potential business investment—did he know of anyone looking for an opportunity? Erick raised his voice and was defensive. He was concerned that someone might take advantage of me financially.

When I told Erick of meeting the recording studio owner, I said, "I get lonely. I miss you. What are you going to do if I have sex with someone else?"

Erick replied, "What can I say? You deserve to not be hidden." He loved and missed me but wished he didn't. *I hoped he'd be jealous and say, "Don't do it."*

Our attachment and bond grew deeper. Right before Christmas, Erick said I was the best present a man could ever want. I desired his warmth, our bodies intertwined. He knew what I meant when I asked him to be with me. *I wanted him to divorce.* When we were together, our love was intimate and pure. We knew each other's likes, wants, and desires and complimented each other professionally. All barriers between us fell away. He breathed life into me and allowed me to be who I am. Our bond was on a different level, beyond 3D—the limited world I had accepted all my life. I said, "When I am with someone else, you are who I think of. I get lonely without you. That is the reason I go out." I wanted to be with just Erick. I knew we could be happy.

When we were together, it was all-consuming and powerful. He could mentally touch me, and I physically felt him. It seemed divine timing was involved. During a moment of intimacy, I told him, "I want you to be in joy and happiness with me forever." I told him I craved him; that I wanted to be inside his body. *To feel his essence.* Our connection would never be replicated. I sensed he felt the same.

On Christmas Eve, Erick came to see me. I gave him a stocking with a few things that wouldn't be noticed. I wanted him to know he was loved. I expected nothing in return. He left my apartment that morning to go shopping. Erick came back while I was napping, and I felt him touch me gently. He had Christmas flowers for me and a couple of gifts similar to what I had given him. He was supposed to have been home for his family celebration, but he stayed longer with me. He didn't want to leave. He was taking an enormous risk, and I worried he might get caught. I knew that on Christmas morning I would be alone and sad. *I was.*

A few days later, Erick was going to a game, and I had plans to go to a live music show. It was freezing in late December, and I almost stayed at home. Erick texted me and his texts made little sense, so I knew he was drinking. He wanted to meet in town to go honky-tonking. I'd never gone bar hopping with live music, so I agreed to join him. He was happy and relaxed. I'm not sure how much he drank, but I saw him drink more. We made our way from bar to bar and danced and sang "Purple Rain." At one point, he spun me to the music—it felt familiar, and I knew it was something we had experienced in a different life. I've never had the ease of dancing with someone in perfect sync. I said, "We have done this before." Although he said nothing, the look on his face seemed to show he recognized it too. I sat close to him and looked into his eyes. He looked at me and said, "People notice you looking at me like I am some kind of God."

We walked outside in the bitter cold with a crowd of people. I felt like we were being watched. I saw a photographer not far away... *Is he photographing us?* I brushed the nagging feeling away. I said, "Be with me, Erick."

He said, "If we were together, most nights would be like this."

At one bar, there was a long lineup of people waiting to gain entry. Erick wanted to see if we could get in—he pulled cash out of his wallet and offered it to the bouncer. It made me uncomfortable; it felt narcissistic. I was glad he was unsuccessful.

Erick wanted us to stay in a hotel that night, but Crystal needed her morning walk, and I replied, "We need to go home." We were both quiet on the ride home. Erick asked me to drop him off in his home driveway, and I said, "No. It's too risky." *I was taken aback. I don't want to be seen.* I couldn't believe he'd asked. Erick had to walk a short distance in the bitter cold to his home at 3:00 a.m. In his words, he was under surveillance. *We had been careless.*

In the new year, Erick flew out of town on business and called me. We texted to break up the monotony of a flight layover and meeting breaks he had. He told me how much he loved me. I made him laugh and smile. I wanted us to be together more and only thought of him when we weren't.

After he was home, we continued feeling each other's energy. It was hard to know who was sending energy first. When I asked if he was sending energy, he said, "You have felt me all day. I miss you." He asked me to go on his upcoming business trip to another state. His intuition is spot on, and he felt we could get away, although there was an element of danger. All that was on his mind was me going with him. I couldn't go to the final destination of his business meeting, but he would drop me at a spa hotel.

Erick arrived early on Thursday, and we started out on the long drive. We were together—that was all that mattered. In the truck, I had a distinct telepathic thought come over me and asked, "Are you thinking about sex?"

He smiled, sheepish, and said, "Yes, I am."

We were in harmony with each other. I performed oral sex as he drove down the interstate.

When I checked in at the spa hotel, they gave me room 222. *Another synchronicity.* I grinned at Erick as I showed him the room number. Angel number 222 offers assurance that things will work out for the best when you focus on your desired outcome, stay positive, and go with the flow. He left after a small amount of alone time with me.

Taking full advantage of the spa, I enjoyed a massage, facial, pedicure, and had my hair styled. We sent energy to each other, and we felt each other's energy. After his meeting, he returned to the hotel late afternoon on Saturday. We were in his truck, and I needed to get something from inside the hotel. Erick said he needed to call Karen and implied it might get loud. As I shut the truck door, I heard yelling. Erick and Karen had a heated argument, and she threatened to come to the hotel, but he didn't think she would show up. That caused me some distress. I didn't ask for details, but he turned his phone off.

We went to a favorite steak restaurant of his. It was nice to not hide and enjoy a romantic meal with him. Erick also wanted to go to a sex toy shop; he wanted to purchase a specific item for me. That night, our pleasure and passion extended to new heights, and I let go fully with him. It was as if I zoned out, feeling everything he did to me without limitations. My mind and body joined his essence, and we were in the moment fully. He asked if I'd had an orgasm because of the way my body reacted to him. He said it was like being in a different dimension, which I couldn't deny. I could only nod yes.

The next morning, Erick was lying on his side, his body curled up on the shower floor, facing the wall as the water rained down upon him. I wanted to lie beside him, but didn't, as I sensed he needed some alone time. I didn't ask questions and lay back down and fell asleep. He woke me up, and we were quiet as we packed our belongings. Our getaway was over. I reached over and played with his arm hair—I couldn't sit right next to him because the console was between us. He grabbed my hand when I stopped, wanting me to continue. I felt that he received little love and affection. It seemed he not only wanted it but craved it. I sensed he dreaded going home and was worried about what would transpire.

After we returned home, Erick texted me. He said his situation was fucked up and wished it wasn't so painful.

I asked, "Does she know?"

"Maybe," he said. "You spoil me."

How long has it been since he's been treated well?

He thanked me for going on the trip with him and said he missed me. I asked him to go with me to the special place we'd created in 5D.

The next morning, Erick asked me to meet him. He told me how tough his evening had been. When he'd arrived home, his best friend and his wife were with Karen. His friend warned Erick that things were bad inside. When Erick had turned his phone off while he was out of town, Karen had called a few people. *She wasn't worried about his safety—she didn't have control over him.* She said, "You wouldn't take my calls, but you talked to V.C. Pitt four times." Each time he'd called me; Karen had known who I was. My anxiety increased.

Erick was drinking to escape what had transpired in his home. We drove by my former marital home, and he questioned how I just walked away. I told him it was no longer my home, and you can if you aren't happy. He said you are like a queen and just do whatever you want. He said I would have to teach him. *Me teach him?*

We drove to my rural childhood town and the surrounding area on a frosty January morning. He learned more about me, and I laughed when he called me Miss Washington County when I gave him the history of landmarks we drove by. He saw my small high school, my childhood homes, and I shared stories about myself. When we drove by Daddy's home, I told Erick stories of what Daddy had done to my immediate family. After telling Erick that Mama discovered Daddy had loosened the lug nuts on her car, he said, "I already don't like him."

We were near Mama's home, and I asked Erick if he wanted to meet her. He was fearful of what she might think because he was married but agreed. I told him she already knew about our situation. He was nice to Mama and handled my stepfather well. In the late evening after we returned to my car, we declared our love. He texted and said the next twenty years were going to be like no other. I should hold on because he was going to rock my world every day for the rest of my life. I was ecstatic.

The next morning, Erick wanted to meet for coffee. I drove to the parking lot we met at the day before and got inside his truck. I noticed a homemade food plate in his truck. I said nothing, but I wondered, *If things are so bad at home, why is there a cooked meal in his vehicle?* We sat down.

"How are things?" I asked. Karen had told him that he could keep his girlfriend, but she wanted to remain married. Things weren't good, but he said Karen was going to attend anger management counseling. I realized this meant he wasn't leaving and said, "Take me back to my vehicle."

He asked, "Can't I finish my coffee?"

I said, "No!"

We drove back in silence. I felt anger rising within me. Before I opened the door, I found my matter-of-fact, eventoned voice and said, "She will continue her behavior. She will not change. DO NOT call me. DO NOT text me." I got out of his truck, shut the door, and didn't look back.

I drove back to my apartment. *What the hell?! Is this a game to him?* In a moment of rage and not thinking my actions through, I changed the area code of his number. I thought I could text, lash out, and press "send," but he wouldn't receive it. I opened our most recent text and typed, "Erick, you are a motherfucker. How dare you hurt me like this? Fuck you. Fuck you. Fuck you, asshole. Why did you even want to see me today? To get your rocks off? Bastard!" I meant every word.

My phone lit up. I felt terrible. I didn't mean for him to receive those words.

He replied, "Of course not. I'm just not good at this, I swear. I put my hand on the Bible." *Meaning, for him, that he was being honest.* "I never want to hurt you. I'd rather spend an eternity in hell than hurt you. Please forgive me. I'm sorry. You know I'm not a 'get my rocks off' kind of guy."

"I needed to release my hurt and anger," I texted.

He felt how angry I was. "Please be patient," he said. "I will be as little of an asshole as I know how to be."

Our texts continued. I apologized for sending hateful messages. *That made me feel shitty...I try not to hurt anyone.* I asked, "Are you working on your marriage, or are you going to be with me?"

Erick replied, "I'm not." He said, "You are lovable."

I said, "You didn't answer my question, and I demand an answer."

He asked if he could tell me later. I said he should tell me if he is working on his marriage. Erick said he was, but didn't know if it would work or not. He didn't want to stop seeing me, but also understood how unfair it was. I felt like someone had punched me in my gut. *I want to hit something, scream, and cry.*

I replied, "That is the answer I needed you to say. We have to stop. This is breaking my heart. I can't keep seeing you. You can't have your cake and eat it too. Don't come to see me. I love you, but you shouldn't have told me you were leaving Karen. If you are working on your marriage, I hope you get what you are looking for. I won't be here if you change your mind a month down the road, but I can't continue to stay like this. Even though you don't think you lied, you did. I feel like a stupid girl, damn you. I'm sorry I can't be all you need me to be. I'm sorry that I won't feel your warmth and kisses again. God, I am so sorry."

I numbed out. I got stoned, stayed high, and sat in my clothes closet, propped up against my clothes washer. As soon as I came down, I smoked more. The pain and anger mixed was horrendous. But I was in shock and couldn't release my emotions.

I numbed out on my closet floor for hours the next day. I was an empty shell, trying to comprehend what had happened. My eyes were red and swollen from crying. Erick texted and asked, "What are you doing?" He was outside looking for me.

"What do you want?"

"Are you fucking kidding?" Erick wanted me now. He came inside.

I was in shambles. I said, "You see the real me." That night, we talked on my closet floor. He went home and he and Karen fought. He told me later that all he could hear was me saying, "She will continue"—and she did. It took a while for me to understand he wanted to be with me. I was scared to believe his words. I couldn't stay mad at him, only love him. Erick wanted to know what we had wasn't just a fling. I accepted him fully and blindly. We didn't make it to bed that night. In the closet, our lovemaking was intense.

The next morning, he went to work. He returned, and there was no drama that evening. We talked about many things, including finding a new church. Erick sat on my black work chair, and I giggled as I wrapped my legs around him as he sang "Green-Eyed Lady" to me. He asked, "Do you promise you will stay with me?"

Immediately, I said, "Yes." He said he wanted to marry me and that I would never have to work again if I didn't want to, not even lift a finger. He had booked a nice vacation with Karen and wondered if he could change the name on the ticket. I remembered that the psychic had mentioned that vacation just two months ago but allowed myself to think about the possibilities of a future with Erick. He walked Crystal with me before bedtime and stayed again that evening. *I could see us getting married on a beach, making love in the mountains, walking hand in hand, riding with the sun's warmth against our skin, sitting on our front porch, together in sickness and in health, just us... I was happy.*

The next morning, he went home to get ready for work. Within thirty minutes, I received a text from Ryan, asking, "How are you?" I then received a text from Erick with verbiage I understood: "Knows and it's bad." *Oh shit!*

"What happened?" I texted back.

"Stay low and keep your doors locked," he said. "I hope I don't get shot. Ryan knows." *Karen told Ryan of our affair because she knew that would hurt Erick. No matter what actions I took, Greg had never told our sons of the affair.* He also said, "Karen was looking for your address in my office." *Holy shit!* She was on her way to their home from his office and was furious. I realized Karen most likely sent the text from Ryan's phone. Erick said, "I'm sorry I got you into this."

"It was me that got you into this," I messaged.

Erick texted: "I'll talk with you later. I'm going dark for a while." My sixth sense was heightened. I was scared, not just for

Erick, but for myself. Although I should have, I hadn't realized what might happen.

Knowing about Karen's previous actions, I knew I had to be cautious. She was everything I wasn't. I stayed inside until late afternoon, not knowing if she would show up at my apartment or try to harm me. Erick had told me she drove a grey Audi. I watched for her car so I wouldn't be surprised if she found me. There were no additional texts from Erick.

Chapter 6

Separation (The Dark Night of the Soul)

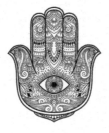

What had happened between Erick and Karen? I watched through slightly open blinds and was careful when walking my dog. I did not receive a text or call from Erick. I needed to be careful. I went to bed fearful.

I texted Erick the following morning and asked, "Are you okay? I'm worried." Wanting to find him, I drove to places I thought he might be. He was outside his office, wearing the same clothes he'd been wearing the day before. He went inside, so I called his office phone: no answer. Someone he worked with arrived, and I drove away. I sent three texts: "Don't retreat into your shell." "Don't shut me out." "I need to know what's happening." No reply.

Later, back at my apartment, I took my garbage outside and saw a grey car driving towards me. *Karen's Audi.* I didn't have my cell phone. *She found me!* Erick had said, "If Karen comes near you, walk the other way." She drove through the warranted no-trespassing parking lot. I got behind some shrubbery. I knew she was looking for me—*what should I do if she confronts me?*

The next day, I checked my email. My stomach turned. There was an email from Karen... *She knows my email address!* In the subject line, she listed a verse from Hebrews 13:4: "Marriage is honourable in all, and the bed undefiled: but whoremongers and adulterers God will judge." (KJV) Her message said, "I thought you might need this. I realized this is your MO. Stay away from Joe.[2] You need to think about what you do. If you value your livelihood you would do what is right in the eyes of the lord."

I shook with anger. Erick had alluded to the fact that Karen doesn't believe in their religion—and now she was trying to use a Bible verse against me! Erick said they had both committed adultery before. I texted a copy of her email to Erick. He needed to know. I wanted him to keep her away from me. *What did he tell her?*

Remembering stories Erick told me about Karen's behavior made me think about who she could be and how volatile their marriage was. Erick said the police had been called to their home on multiple occasions.

When things had erupted between them, Erick had left their home to stay in a hotel. He had told me that Karen had locked him out of their home. Varying thoughts popped into my mind about intimate details that Erick shared.

---

[2] "Joe" was a mutual colleague of mine and Erick's. For some reason, Karen had surmised that I was having an affair with Joe, who was a married—I was not. Our relationship was strictly professional.

Erick felt that only one of his friends might be upset if they were to separate. By Erick's own admission, he would've taken a bullet for Karen at one time, but not anymore. Although I didn't personally witness the things he told me, I believe Erick's account fully. I thought about the time I saw them at a store and how uncomfortable I felt towards her.

Why does someone stay in an unhappy and controlling situation? *I couldn't.* An abuser can make the victim think everything is their fault. My belief is he was conditioned over the years to accept emotional abuse that he now accepts as normal behavior.

Knowing Erick had an upcoming appointment at a local clinic, I drove there and watched for him to return to his vehicle. He walked to his vehicle and seemed okay. I rolled the window down and said his name. He looked at me, clenched his jaw, and looked around the parking lot. He drove away. I sat there, in shock and disbelief. He'd ghosted me! Driving home, I was mad and hurt. I borrowed someone's phone and sent him a text: "You could have at least said goodbye." Erick turned his back on me. I was spent. Never in my wildest dreams did I see any of this happening. That night, I numbed out in my closet. Email notifications showed Karen was viewing my social media profile. The last week had taken an emotional toll on me. I was a walking corpse.

My grief continued. I was nervous and inconsolable. There were no words to express the heartache I experienced. Two weeks after the affair was exposed, I found part of my Christmas gift to him underneath my vehicle's windshield wipers. At first, I thought Erick had returned it, but I realized he didn't return a few other small gifts, so it must have been Karen. It scared me knowing that Karen had returned the gift while I slept less than fifteen feet away. Underneath my SUV, I found plastic tubing with enclosed wires that appeared to have been pulled from the undercarriage. *She doesn't want to just scare me...she might want to harm me!* I had security cameras installed to protect myself.

Karen sent a second email with the subject line of "whore." She said I was a "slut bitch wannabe home Wreaker!" (*sic*) But all I had done, she said, was to make her husband love her more. "You are a giant piece of SHIT! Never try to contact him, even with someone else's phone. Yes, he told me you did."

"He finds you totally repulsive. You slimy bitch. Your ex-husband is very fortunate to be rid of your nasty ass!" *Her spelling, wording, and punctuation skills are lacking.* I didn't want to face the fact that Erick wouldn't be back.

I was living in fear and filed a police report for harassment. After I left the police station, I knew Erick would have his weekly appointment nearby and park in a public lot. Having copies of the emails, I made a split decision to leave them on his windshield with a handwritten note: "She needs to leave me alone. I reported her to the police." I kept my distance and watched Erick walk to his vehicle and retrieve the copies. Maybe I am naïve or disillusioned, but I never saw it all playing out as it did.

When I notified my apartment manager about the harassment and the circumstances of my situation, she asked me to speak with an officer who lived in our complex. He gave me no sympathy, saying, "Marriage is still recognized in this state." I told him I'd contacted a report officer (with whom I'd left copies of the emails), I'd left a note on Erick's windshield, I wouldn't be contacting either of them, and that I expected the same.

Karen sent a third email with the subject "police report." Both of them had filed reports as well, she said. "Erick told law enforcement about you calling from another line and that you left emails on his vehicle. Stay the fuck away!" Her emails were degrading. I didn't call him—I'd only *texted* from another phone. The situation consumed me. Karen was terrorizing me.

Immersed in what author Eckhart Tolle refers to as "the pain body,"[3] I was on a downward spiral, losing bits of myself. Tears, sadness, hopelessness, depression, and darkness were with me all the time. I began seeing my therapist again. It helped to talk about it, but I never allowed myself to have a breakthrough—I saw crying in front of others as weakness.

One afternoon, two of my co-workers and I worked in my apartment. Near the end of the day, one mentioned seeing a vehicle with a woman inside who had been there most of the day. We talked about it. Samantha was there and had noticed the vehicle, too. I'd felt like I was being watched, but we didn't talk about it or piece it together until later in the day. *Did Karen have someone watching me?* Karen left me a voice message saying, "Quit being a chickenshit. Call me." My anxiety skyrocketed. My depression medication stopped working.

The property manager called me; she had received a voice message, a complaint, from someone named Sally Justin who had visited a friend at the apartment complex. Sally's message said, "It's a family community. There was a powerful presence of pot coming from apartment number 369, and there was a lot of it coming and going from that apartment." *Sally and Karen sounded identical.* Although I smoked pot, I took every precaution, including using an air purifier, so no one could smell it. The people "coming and going" from my apartment were the five women I worked with. The manager liked me and agreed that it was Karen who had called. The manager knew of women like her, and she decided to put Karen in her place. She made a return phone call to "Sally" in my presence, but there was no answer. The manager gave me a copy of the message.

---

[3] Tolle, Eckhart. *The Power of Now: A Guide to Spiritual Enlightenment.* Vancouver, BC. Namaste Publishing. 1999. Print.
Tolle, Eckhart. *The Power of Now: A Guide to Spiritual Enlightenment.* Novato, California. New World Library. 2000. Audio.

The voice message sounded like Karen, and I wrote the number down and put it aside.

I was furious that she was trying to get me evicted from my apartment. *If she thinks I'm moving, she's wrong. Does she feel threatened by me living so close to her and Erick?* After I thought about it and pieced it together, I questioned if Karen may have hired someone to watch my place. I will never know. I will also never know if she hired someone to photograph us on the night we went honky-tonking—but in my gut, I believe she did.

At that point, I knew Erick had used the story we had discussed if Karen discovered the affair: We'd agreed that he would tell her we'd smoked pot together and that one thing led to another. I wondered: *Did he blame me? Did he take any responsibility?* He had been bullied in the past. She thought she could do the same to me. *If I was evicted and moved, I wouldn't be a threat any longer.*

I received calls from a strange phone number, and an online search showed they were from a phone app. I traveled out of town for a work conference, and twice in one afternoon, the same phone number came in on my phone. Something about the number alerted my intuition. When I got home, I located the number I'd put aside. My heart raced—it was the same number as the calls to the apartment complex. I told the police I thought Karen was retaliating for me contacting them.

I remember Erick and I were together and discussed what we would do if our affair was ever found out. He said that if Greg came near him or his family, he would damn near kill him. I replied that if Karen came near me, I would go to the police. It seemed Erick had done nothing to stop her. I wanted to tell him. With her threatening behavior increasing, I couldn't wrap my head around everything that was happening. I hadn't fired my gun in a while, so I took a private defensive class. I learned to shoot by holding the gun in each hand, in case I had to defend myself.

One weekday, with co-workers present, I walked my dog outside the apartment complex. For months, my ears had buzzed twenty-four hours a day, seven days a week. The pitch changed, which got my attention. I looked straight ahead and saw Karen's Audi in my parking lot. Nervous, I reached into my pocket for my cell phone. *It's not there. It's inside my apartment. Is she going to confront me? Intimidate me? What should I do?* She drove around the parking lot. My security camera caught her, and I contacted the police again. My world was imploding. Anxiety-ridden, I slept little, couldn't focus, and was always on the brink of tears.

A few mornings later, I woke up early and walked Crystal. I had my gun on me, but I wasn't as observant as usual. I saw a car speeding toward me, revving the engine. *Karen's Audi?* Tired of what I perceived as increased threats, I called the police. The officer said, "The next person who makes contact will be in trouble."

I said, "I haven't contacted either of them, other than what I have told you. It's a shame that you won't do anything about her actions." *Are you fucking kidding me?!*

He told me that when he'd asked if she'd called me from a phone app, she denied it. She told him she is sometimes in my area, going to a movie with Ryan. Disgusted, I worried her threats might increase.

The officer called me back later to say he had found the owner of the number who called me. Since nothing else had gone in my favor, I thought he'd say it wasn't Karen. He'd called the number, and she had answered. "Do you want to press charges?" he asked.

"Yes." I felt vindicated. The police filed a report against Karen for harassment on my behalf, which went to the district attorney's office. She would have to turn herself in to law enforcement. Police vehicles sat in a nearby parking lot in the mornings. *The police realized she might try to hurt me.*

I breathed a sigh of relief when I saw on a website that Karen had been booked at the county jail, charged with harassment. The General Sessions subpoena arrived with a court date. The DA would represent me. A continuance was granted, and they pushed the court date out.

I was paranoid. My gut told me I needed to search my name online. I found a negative website review of me from someone Karen's age, who lived in the same town. I contacted the website, and the comment was removed. I was angry that she kept rattling my cage and trying to intimidate me. But all I could do was wait for court.

Greg hadn't told our kids about the affair. Worrying they might find out about the restraining order or that Karen might try to contact them, I was honest and disclosed to Kurt and Roman (who were twenty-four and eighteen at the time) what had happened. When I asked Kurt if he hated me, he shrugged his shoulders, turned his back on me, and walked away. I gave him space, let the truth soak in, and give him time to forgive me. When I told Roman, he gave me a hug and said, "I love you Mom." I had expected an opposite reaction.

I was trying to find a new normal. I saw Angel numbers more frequently. About this time, I started pulling my tarot cards for insight into the court situation. The Justice card came out repeatedly. It was related to the upcoming court date, which implied that justice would be served. *Does this mean that Karen will get justice or I will?* Signs and synchronicities continued. *I still see Erick's name and initials everywhere.* Samantha signed me up on a couple of dating websites, but I wasn't ready. I was matched daily to men named "Erick," spelled multiple ways, and men who were business coaches like Erick.

I found an older newspaper with Roman listed as student of the month, and on the same page was a residential home advertisement for the complex in which Erick's grandmother had lived. *More than coincidence.*

Before Erick had ghosted me, we'd created our special place in 5D. Erick told me how much he loved the Blue Ridge Mountains and told me how beautiful they were. *I want to see them.* He had wanted us to travel by train car and make love on an overlook in those mountains. *I had wanted that, too. To make love in God's country.* Our vision had stayed with me. I hired someone to paint the image. When I saw it, it wasn't as I'd fully imagined it—the overlook and mountains were missing, and instead of a creek, a stream was on the canvas—but I liked the finished illustration. I hung it over my bed.

Court was postponed again until June. *Ugh.* As the date neared, I felt anxious about facing Karen. *Will Erick be by her side?* Samantha was my support system and agreed to go to court with me. Aunt Lauren, a special aunt of mine, gave me courage and wisdom for the situation.

Waiting until right before the court's roll call, I walked in and sat down, not realizing I was only five rows behind Erick and Karen. I wanted to vomit. When my name was called, I couldn't find my voice and raised my hand. Erick turned to find me. His face was deep-red—his blood pressure was extremely high. Karen looked at me. Samantha and I saw Erick look back at me two more times. I felt nauseous. I wanted to run out of the courtroom, but to feel safe again, I needed a restraining order.

Karen walked to the back of the room. She smirked and tried to intimidate me. I stared into her eyes. I didn't look away. If she wanted me to cower, she got no satisfaction. I wanted to inflict harm, but that is not who I am. I blocked my energetic connection with Erick. As he walked out of the room, he looked at the ground. His face was still crimson. *Is he going to stroke out?* The clothes he was wearing had hung on my bedroom door in the early mornings we'd shared. I thought, "You asshole," and hoped he received it telepathically.

When the DA representative approached me, she asked me to step outside to discuss my complaint. She stopped in front of where Erick and Karen were sitting. Both were listening to what the DA was telling me. They were laughing and smiling on the wooden bench together. Disgusted, I asked the DA to move our conversation to a different area. She asked for details of my evidence. "What do you want?" she asked.

"A restraining order and reimbursement on my security cameras," I said.

There was a high case volume that day, and the DA told me she might not be able to stand with me when the case was called. Panicked, I felt an anxiety attack coming on. As I sat in the courtroom, my foot tapped and my right knee bounced. Samantha placed her hand on my knee to stop the noise. I wanted the proceedings to be over.

Karen's criminal attorney asked what evidence I had. I had a folder containing the three emails she'd sent me, copies of social media emails showing Karen's repeated views, photos of the wiring pulled from my vehicle and the gift left under my windshield, and a record of the phone app numbers that had called. I said I had cell phone footage of her going through my warranted no-trespassing parking lot, a cell phone recording of her telling me to quit being a chickenshit and call her, and the voice message in which she tried to get me kicked out of my apartment.

He read the emails, and his eyes opened wide. "What do you want?" he asked.

"A restraining order and reimbursement for my security cameras," I said. My anger spilled out, and in a deep voice through my clenched jaw, I said, "I want her to leave me alone! To leave me alone! To leave me alone!"

Karen and Erick stayed out of the courtroom most of the day. The DA said that Karen's attorney had agreed to a six-month restraining order and reimbursement for my security cameras. I should have been satisfied with the agreement, but I was upset that they had forced me to be on display. I took a half of a Xanax to take the edge off my anxiety. I was in the middle of my own shit storm. I wanted off of this merry-go-round, but without being thrown off.

Karen returned to the courtroom, looking unconcerned. Erick wasn't with her, and I realized later that he'd gone to get a check to pay for my security cameras. It was a messed-up situation. I was paying for our sins emotionally. He was paying for his indiscretion with money. I wanted her to pay for my security cameras, not him, but Karen had made him reconcile his affair in multiple ways. The cost of a retainer for a criminal attorney was high—it would have been a few thousand dollars (in addition to the hourly rate). We were in court for several hours. Karen and her attorney approached the bench. The DA and I did the same. I had to walk by Erick and felt him looking at me. The attorneys had already agreed, but we still were required to stand before the judge. The judge read Karen's charge of harassment. I was relieved he didn't state the reasons for her charge.

Karen and I stood three feet from each other. The judge issued a "strong" restraining order against Karen—she was to act as if I had fallen off the face of the earth and have no contact with me. She chimed in, "No worries there." *It was a game for her!*

The DA handed me the check with my name on it and Erick as the remitter for reimbursement on my security cameras. The judge looked at me and said, "If Karen contacts or approaches you, call the police or my office."

I said, "Thank you, Your Honor." I turned around, hoping my hand would stop shaking so I could turn the handle on the short gate separating me from the audience. Neither Erick nor I looked at each other, but I closed the gate and sent a "Fuck you for making me do this" thought to him telepathically.

Samantha and I left the courtroom. I wanted to forget everything that had transpired. Drained, I was about to cry. Samantha drove me home, and we passed a stop light where

Erick's truck was idling. I'm not sure if they saw us. *Oh my God, please let me disappear.* Back at home, inside my closet on the floor, I numbed out for the rest of the evening. I cried. I was lost and in soul shock. Living an inescapable nightmare, the events replayed in my mind. *Erick doesn't care. He's betrayed me. I'm gentle and wasn't created to have my broken heart trampled on. No words or emotions are left. I am empty. A shell of who I was five months ago. How am I going to live; get past this?* My dark night of the soul continued for weeks.

Chapter 7
Connection Through Synchronicity

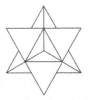

No matter how I tried, I couldn't find my footing in life after court. The pain body was horrendous. It consumed me. I was being pulled into a dark abyss, treading water. I couldn't swim to shore. That remains the most difficult period in my life. It brought me to my knees. My tears were unending. Trying to run a successful business was overwhelming. I felt lost.

In a little over a year, I'd had a spiritual awakening and an all-consuming affair. I'd divorced, moved, and been harassed. Kurt wasn't speaking to me. He wouldn't respond to my calls or texts. I never thought he would reject me, but he did. I'd gone through harassment, court proceedings, and had lost Erick. My joy and happiness had evaporated. I was anxious and hadn't smiled in weeks. One night, I hit a low point. I knew I shouldn't be alone, so Samantha stayed with me. No amount of numbing out would help me—I realized I might drown in my dark abyss. Samantha saved me from myself that night.

Samantha and I flew to stay with her family in Colorado. Colorado is beautiful and offered me the beginning stages of healing. The scenery and snow-capped mountains were majestic, even at the end of June. I sat by a lake, and the nature surrounding me helped me see God's beauty on a larger scale. I smiled, felt peaceful, and looked at the puffy clouds. I saw a unicorn fill a section of the vast sky. Erick and I had a running joke that I was "a unicorn." Late one afternoon, a double rainbow came over the mountains. I felt hopeful.

I wondered, *How far am I from home?* I did a search. Synchronistically, the number of miles was Erick's street address number. One night, Erick came to me in a dream. I heard his voice say, "Don't sleep with anyone else."

I visited small shops in town the following day. There was a crystal and stone jewelry shop that I was drawn to. A rhodochrosite necklace drew me in. The stone is for compassion and enhances positivity while stimulating the release of unresolved emotional pain. A protective mystic topaz ring caught my eye—topaz possesses healing properties while releasing depression, fear, and anxiety. I purchased both, and they became favorite pieces I wore daily for months. Although far from happy, after flying home, I took a step forward.

I continued to see repetitive Angel numbers that gave me messages— everything from 111, 333, 555, 777, and mirroring numbers—I found peace and comfort in them. *The messages mean I was manifesting, Angels are with me, and changes are coming.* I saw the last four digits of Erick's cell number on license plates and when shopping and making purchases. Dating websites continued to make suggestions for connections with men named Erick, Erik, or Eric. Many matches were business coaches. Erick's name appeared on TV, in business ads, in YouTube videos, in news articles, and in online stories. Movie credits included references to people named Erick and his profession.

Close friends tried to be supportive. Everyone around me seemed to have normal, happy relationships. Still melancholy, I listened to spiritual readers and tried to get as much information on the Internet regarding mirroring between Twin Flames as possible. I learned twins can mirror childhood wounds and adult traumas. I realized it would need to be me who raised my internal vibration and frequency to help both Erick and myself.

I am a Divine Feminine, and Erick is my Divine Masculine. Online searches will give you many explanations. I learned everyone has masculine and feminine traits; for example, some people are intuitive (a feminine trait), and some people are logical (a masculine trait).[4] It is up to each of one of us to get a balance of both energies. I realized I have been in my masculine energy for well over twenty years, and that I had to heal my wounds and traumas, and make energetic changes within me.

My ability to engage in sexuality with sensuality resulted from me having been with Erick. I have been told this is part of my essence, which I embrace. Divine Masculines trigger it within the Divine Feminines. We weren't together, but I felt Erick sexually and energetically. I felt anxiety I knew wasn't mine: Erick was having a difficult time. Some nights I woke up with severe anxiety. *Are these Erick's emotions or mine?* My face would turn red and be hot on different occasions when my energy was calm. I believe I absorb Erick's anxiety and high blood pressure when this happens. *It continues to happen three years later.*

I had a dream about Erick and Karen and another about him and a former co-worker. I didn't know what the dream represented. Over the weeks and months that followed, multiple synchronicities happened. I saw Erick's name and initials, his date of birth, his family members' names, his animals' names, and repeated number sequences. My intuition kept bringing

---

[4] https://beyondtheordinaryshow.com/spiritual-dictionary/divine-balance-masculine-feminine/

me back to Erick's sister's death many years ago. He had only said that an accident claimed her life and that they were close. I remembered the sadness in his voice when he told me the story. To marry on the anniversary of a loved one's death—he must have been tormented. *What had happened all those years ago?* I couldn't find the information online, but a small community library directed me to a larger metropolitan public library.

A librarian in the archives section assisted me and found the obituaries of two names I searched. She printed copies for me. Inside a room with large metal filing cabinets, there were hundreds of microfiche containing scans of older newspapers. I remembered Erick's sister's death date but was unsure of the year. My gut told me to try one particular year, and I started reviewing pages of the newspaper. I found it on the second roll of microfiche within an hour. I couldn't believe my eyes—I'd found a needle in a haystack. *OMG... He and I were the same age, six months apart, when Brian almost died in a car wreck. Our siblings were one year apart in age when the accidents happened.*

I read the article and felt sad about the accident which had caused his family to implode. Something within me wanted to go to visit the cemetery. The obituaries showed that his sister and father are buried there. I found four of his family's graves side by side. I saw synchronicities that weren't in my imagination. Erick's father's birthday was my close cousin's birthday and his death day was my birthday. The synchronicity seemed more profound when I remembered the specific birthday on which Erick's father had died—it was the night a train had almost hit me. Erick's grandfather's death day was my Grandpa's birthday, but a different year. His grandmother's name was identical to my second great-aunt's name. There were so many dates on which important events had occurred for both of us. For example, as I looked at his grandmother's death date, I recalled I had been trying to conceive my oldest child on that day. As I stood in the graveyard examining the headstones, I realized my clairsentience had led me to do the research at the library, which led to me being a sleuth at the graveyard and finding the information—*was I supposed to discover it?* This cemented my inner knowledge that Erick and I were Twin Flames. Twins have synchronicity with dates, names, and addresses in their families which are beyond coincidence, and there were astronomical odds that there would be this many synchronicities between us.

I found Erick's favorite grandmother's obituary online. I held my breath when I found two synchronicities: One of the memorial notations referenced that instead of flowers, mourners should contribute to the Shriners' organization. Kurt was a patient of Shriners a few years ago, and they had performed an expensive, helpful complex jaw surgery that was not covered on his medical insurance. I remembered Erick had mentioned his grandfather was a Shriner before my business started. *My step-father was a Shriner, too.*

Years ago, Erick's grandmother had worked in the same place as my Aunt Lauren—at a large engineering company in town. I asked Aunt Lauren if she knew her. She worked there at the same time and described her to me. I shook my head—another synchronicity!

All the signs and synchronicities I was receiving made me wonder: *Is it time to contact Erick?* I had always found peace at the lake he and I had visited. I needed time to myself, so I went. I saw a can of Erick's favorite brand of beer on the small dock. I went within.

I purchased a burner phone and messaged him. I sent a text with cryptic information that only he could interpret and no one else would understand. "I'm childlike not wanting to be betrayed & stroking my hair knowing I'm in a different dimension dancing in the purple rain while eating mashed potatoes & sugarloaf at an overlook seeing 1111 wildflowers in a field hearing the loud waterfalls." No response. Two weeks later, I sent a message of spiritual references and hoped it would help him on his journey. "Divine timing, synchronicities, spirituality, faith, telepathy, connection. Raise internal vibration and must heal childhood wounds/addictions. DM/DF energy and traits must balance in both."

A week later, on Christmas morning, I awoke from a dead sleep—in my dream, Erick and I were kissing. I felt him connecting with me through astral travel or in 5D. It felt so real and intimate. It was reminiscent of him wrapping the Harry Potter scarf around my face and kissing me. I longed for him. His energy was undeniable. The following week, I sent a third message and included a photo of the 5D painting. At the end of the message I typed, "If you don't want me to send you anything else, text stop." Two minutes later, I received a reply: "Stop." *Are we really on a Twin Flame journey?*

Another dark night of the soul brought me to my knees. I prayed and sought spiritual guidance. I pushed through the next week. *He is the Twin Flame runner, and I'm the chaser.* A Gulf beach getaway would allow me to work on my healing and detach from Erick's energy. I booked a trip to Orange Beach with family and friends for January. When we arrived, I couldn't wait to get my feet in the ocean. I rolled up my jeans and walked into the rough waves. Much-needed joy inflamed my heart. As enormous waves crashed into me, I laughed.

I stayed alone a substantial part of the time. Wanting to try something new, I booked a session of salt float therapy. Spending time in a pitch-black chamber filled with salt water, I adapted to the sensory deprivation. I sought knowledge in the tank from Spirit and the Universe—but wasn't successful.

Back at the condo, I sat on the balcony and prayed that I could release Erick and separate from his energy. I looked into the sky, praying, relaxing my mind, and seeking guidance and answers. Gold spots and flecks formed a mystical, geometrical pattern above me. It's the result of two opposing tetrahedrons being joined. These tetrahedrons spun in opposite directions. It was both spiritual and supernatural. I discovered later it was a three-dimensional Star of David known as a Merkabah, a sacred geometry symbol. The Merkabah is a 3D energy field which provides protection and transports your consciousness into higher dimensions. It combines opposing energies, resulting in perfect masculine and feminine energies. I thanked God for being part of that powerful moment.

At the beach, combining the Merkabah with the full moon's intense, deep emotional energy invigorated me. *It's powerful!* I had traveled almost 500 miles to release Erick's energy. But I wasn't ready. He had texted the word "Stop." I needed to move away from his energy. Before lunch, I relaxed my mind and let it wander. I remembered happy, tender, sad, and painful moments. Our laughter, passionate kisses, and supportive conversations bubbled to the surface. I remembered meeting Erick, not being able to pinpoint what I felt. He had believed in me, he had guided me, he had triggered my spiritual awakening. Our sexual liaison had become an intense affair—and together we had known deep love. I remembered seeing his face morph, the long nights of separation and longing after the affair ended, my harassment, the court proceedings, the Christmas morning kiss that woke me, and him rejecting me with the word "Stop."

I spoke to Erick telepathically. "I didn't know what true love was before I met you," I told him. "You are my muse. I have to let you go, but I don't want to. It is painful but necessary." As strange as it may seem, I felt like he heard me. Our connection transcends time and miles. On the white sand, I looked into the sky seeking peace, wanting to stop the aching and indescribable pain of missing the other half of my soul. Other twins understand emptiness and longing. I missed everything about him, from his laugh and sense of humor to the words he said to me when we were together, to his kisses, his passion for me, and the vulnerability and deep connection we shared.

That day was exhausting. I lay face down on my bed, cried, and thought of Erick. I began feeling what I can only describe as his energetic presence. I felt his stomach on my back and the familiar feeling of his body against mine while having sex. I felt his energy protesting me walking away from him and the connection we shared—and I knew he could merge with my energy 500 miles away since we felt each other while I was 175 miles away. I felt intense passion and what I refer to as "twinergetic love" where one body begins and the other ends. Erick's energy was powerful. *Supernatural.*

I remained alone for three additional nights at the beach. One night, I slept on the balcony with a light blanket. I kept the doors open and took in every bit of salty air and cool sand I could. I felt more peace than I have in a year.

When it was time to go home, I made one last gesture of releasing Erick's energy. I was on the beach and drew several words in the sand with a stick, including the word "unconditional."

I watched the waves wash them away. As I drove, I listened to *The Power of Now* audio by Eckhart Tolle,[5] which Erick had recommended. Along the way, I passed many license plates, billboards, and Angel numbers, beginning with 111, 222, 333, etcetera. I had done all I could to release Erick.

After my return home, Erick's rejection set in. I obsessed over recent events and spiraled out of control. For the first time, I became angry at Erick and numbed out. Hoping he felt a fraction of the pain he had caused me, I wanted to hurt him.

An attractive professional man on an adult dating site named Brice sent me a message at a vulnerable time. Brice came to my apartment for a fling, and I was in my full-blown

---

[5] Tolle, Eckhart. *The Power of Now: A Guide to Spiritual Enlightenment.* Vancouver, BC. Namaste Publishing. 1999. Print.
Tolle, Eckhart. The Power of Now: A Guide to Spiritual Enlightenment. Novato, California. New World Library. 2000. Audio.

sexuality. I had revenge sex with him—something I'd never done. I tried to replicate what I felt with Erick.

I knew Erick felt my sexual energy because our connection exists even when we are separated. Feeling the anger boiling inside me, I asked Brice if he would use a toy—he seemed happy to oblige. Knowing that Erick felt me when I was having sex, I disconnected from Brice and linked to Erick. My body went through the motions. While I emotionally disconnected from Brice, I called Erick telepathically. *"Another man is using the toy you bought me. I hope you feel every thrust."* I gave him a psychic play-by-play of what was happening. It was vengeful, angry sex.

It took two days for me to realize the full weight of my actions. I went to Walmart during the Super Bowl half-time show and thought I saw Erick in the parking lot at the same time—*had he seen me?* Seeing him, I felt rejection, bitterness, and rage rising up in me. The way I'd felt made me realize I didn't like myself. As I stewed about who I'd become, I felt remorse. I dropped to my knees when I returned home, asking God to forgive me.

Over the next few days, I prayed and tried to make amends with Erick through telepathy. Disgusted with myself, I asked him psychically and multiple times to forgive me. Soon after, I tried to locate my self-respect and began reconnecting with who I truly am.

Chapter 8

Soulmate Recognition

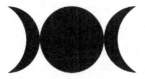

In January, a year had passed since Erick had ghosted me. I was attending a class at a local club, and the instructor mentioned a risqué website for singles. Curious, I joined. I received a message from Chris, who intrigued me. His spirituality was appealing, and he seemed to understand me. Our communication was via the web, which increased my level of comfort.

We agreed to meet at a local sports bar on a Sunday morning in late January. Chris told me he would greet me at the corner of the restaurant with a soulful kiss, which made me nervous—but I couldn't wait to meet him. The restraining order had expired, and I was still worried about running into Erick and Karen. So, to protect myself against a possible uncomfortable situation arising, I said, "If I ask you, 'Is the sky blue?' will you leave, no questions asked?"

"Of course," Chris assured me.

On Sunday, I wore a sleeveless black and white dress with a black leather jacket and boots. When I arrived at the sports bar, I walked a little faster than normal. I saw Chris waiting. He was wearing a dressy hat, a dark sports jacket, and a light-colored dress shirt with pressed jeans and nice boots. He stands

5'10", is bald, and has a neatly trimmed, long mustache on his handsome face. He greeted me with a huge smile. I walked over to him, and he took me in his arms with a warm embrace and gave me that soulful kiss he'd promised. People on the busy street corner saw us. I was fearless.

After being seated, we ordered drinks and our conversation flowed. Chris smiled at me and asked, "Is the sky blue?"

Looking up at the bright sunshine against the blue canvas sky, I smiled. "No," I said.

We enjoyed getting to know each other. He was looking for "her" and wanted to love and cherish that person. I wanted to learn more about him. I was a little lit after a few drinks. Chris told me I would crave many things, emotionally and sexually, in the upcoming days. Through BDSM, he would mark me emotionally. I was skeptical, but I realize the bond is strong between a Dominant and a submissive. I lived a half-mile away, and he offered to follow me home in his truck to make sure I made it. I agreed and invited him to come in.

Still feeling the effects of the drinks, I felt brave. Testing the waters, I surprised myself—I bent over a chair, propped myself on the arm of the chair, and looked at him seductively. We fooled around but without full intimacy. It felt familiar between us. After a few hours, he gave me a deep kiss and left. I wanted more time together.

We exchanged cell numbers and communicated more, and I anticipated our next date eagerly. Thinking about Chris helped me to not focus so much on Erick. He picked me up in his clean, oversized truck. We hadn't planned a full date, but I knew we were going to the Harley Davidson store and stopping at the Hustler store. He is a longtime motorcycle rider, which gives him freedom. I admire that he finds inner peace when riding. He took me to two dealerships and asked my opinion on bikes. Chris was looking for "her"—and I realized that instead of purchasing a motorcycle and then connecting with "her," he wanted to find "her" and then make a purchase. This scared me a little, as I wasn't sure I would be the "her" he was seeking.

We left the dealership, and I knew where our next stop would be. I became a little anxious. Getting acquainted on the website as we did, I knew part of our outing would include going to a sex-toy retail store that makes most people blush.

I walked inside. I was inquisitive about how the different products worked. Looking at merchandise, we went to a specific section. We both agreed on a flogger and purchased it. *Am I going to do this? Yes, I am.* With Chris being a Dominant, I wasn't sure what to expect. I was nervous, but onboard for whatever would transpire.

I loved flogging. I was glad I'd met a Dom who understood my wants and needs. I had to decide if I could be a submissive.

Over the next few weeks, I researched being submissive and was overwhelmed by the different terms related to this type of relationship. A Dominant/submissive relationship involves much more than was depicted in the movie *50 Shades of Grey*. The relationship is a power exchange and involves both parties giving consent and drawing boundaries—those issues weren't fully addressed in the movie.

I knew that if anyone ever tried to hurt me, Chris would do them harm. We had many conversations revolving around us and the possibility *and probability* of me becoming submissive. Contrary to what you might think, a submissive is one of the strongest people you will ever meet. A submissive gives up control, but that person gets a lot in return from the Dom, for as noted, it's a power exchange. Chris wanted to love and cherish "her." It was up to me whether I was strong enough to relinquish control to him.

My texts and talks with Chris provided me with happiness and a familiarity I hadn't experienced since Erick. I looked forward to being with him. But Erick's ghost still haunted me, and his energy stayed with me. Once I mentioned to Chris that I was a Twin Flame and I told him about an affair that had defined me. It was wrong to not tell him the full story up front. Even though he is spiritual, I thought he wouldn't understand. I didn't want to disappoint him. The further we went into our relationship, the less likely I was to tell him. One night while making love with Chris, I felt Erick's energy. This had happened once before when I'd had revenge sex, and intuitively, I knew Erick could feel when I was being intimate with someone.

I tried to ignore that Chris and Erick shared similarities. Both are smokers; they like the same college football team; love to fish and wear fishing shirts; have the same favorite color; drive the same color large trucks; and like Westerns. They both think of John Wayne as their hero. Later, I discovered that both of them also like the same food and beverages. I wondered: *Is this coincidence or synchronicity? Is the Universe playing a trick on me or comforting me with familiarity?*

Chris has a distinct and desirable body. He has broad shoulders, with a small waist and hips, like the letter V. It made me wonder why he found me attractive since I am a plus size, but I never questioned it—he always made me feel desired. One night while we texted, I envisioned a different time. *I saw him through my third eye.* He was inside a pyramid; there was a torch on the wall. In the torch's light, I saw him wearing the white clothing of an Egyptian ruler, with a Nemes *headdress*. He wore black kohl around his eyes. That image is still strong in my mind's eye. He commented that I may have served him then.

In the passing days, we talked more about spirituality. Chris gets visions through dreams, which fascinates me—it differs from my spiritual gifts. I told Samantha, "Things are natural and easy between us." The next day, Chris used the same words to describe our relationship. He felt that a higher power had orchestrated our meeting. I came to the same conclusion: *We are soulmates.*

Once, I went by his work for a tour of the enormous building he oversees. He introduced me to his coworkers. His work impressed me. After the tour, he walked me to my car. I shocked myself when he kissed me goodbye and "I lov—" escaped my lips. I tried to recover. My heart was pounding. I hoped he didn't realize my Freudian slip—and I'm not sure whom it surprised more. We texted later, and it didn't get by him after all—"Good recovery," he said. *How did this happen? I wasn't supposed to fall in love with him.* It felt like I was betraying my twin, but I was happy when Chris said, "I love you."

Sometimes I find peace at the lake. While lying on the small dock where I had seen Erick's favorite beer-can brand, I cried and asked God, Spirit, and the Universe, *Give me clarification. Am I supposed to move away from my twin?* Deep in thought and almost meditative, I heard my first channeled song, "Just to Be Close to You" by the Commodores. As I looked into the sky, I saw a cloud that formed an Angel shape with Erick's facial features. Within ten minutes of leaving, I saw Erick's date of birth on a license plate and the Angel number 111. The temperature was his birth year, and I saw his initials on the side of a truck in a parking lot. When I ordered dinner, the total bill equaled Erick's street address. *Synchronicity.*

Chris and I became closer and one day, a text conversation we had triggered core wounds within me. Chris had shared an afternoon with someone famous years ago, and my self-worth wound was triggered, which caused immediate anxiety. The rush of emotion made me feel inadequate, and anxiety overcame me. I wanted to run. Chris had plans that afternoon, but he felt he needed to come to me and talk. I knew I had to be vulnerable and open up to him, although I was hesitant. He was loving and kind to me—he treated me like a queen. I didn't understand why, nor felt I deserved it.

Before Chris came over, I started drinking vanilla rum and coke. I couldn't tell him my deepest feelings without a little liquid courage. He arrived and was patient with me while I explained my core wounds. Most everyone has wounds that carry over from childhood into adulthood. Mine are rejection, abandonment, and lack of self-worth. I felt unworthy because I saw photos online of the woman he'd shared time with—I felt I was less than her. Sitting on his lap like a child, I was afraid to be open with him. He soothed me, and I told him about the times men had rejected me. By being open with him, I experienced healing. It wasn't painful. I told him I would answer his questions about my Twin Flame affair later. My love for him deepened.

During this time, I found a new house I wanted to buy. My financial obligation of paying Greg's house payment had ended. With Chris' background in commercial buildings, I asked him to assist me in build-out decisions for my new home, and he did. I was excited to make color and flooring choices. It would be what I wanted.

As I became more spiritually connected, I practiced manifestation and release during moon cycles. I started feeling my internal vibration increase. That powerful feeling was partially because of Chris' strength, which carried over to me. On April 7, I looked up at the full moon and said to the Universe, "I am ready for whatever you want me to do."

The Universe was waiting for that statement. A week later, the wheels were in motion for events for which I was unprepared. On April 13, the horrible manager I dealt with at work chose to ignore my solid recommendations. If I had planted my feet firmly on the ground (as I normally did), I would have lost a contract and would have had to terminate the contractors who worked with me. I thought outside the box and salvaged the contract.

On April 14, an adult neighbor from my childhood named Eric reached out to me. Daddy had called him thinking Eric could convince me to call him. Three years earlier, I had pulled away from Brian and Daddy because of their toxicity and how it affected me and no longer communicated with them. It irritated me that Daddy played on someone's sympathies to have them reach out to me. He knew I thought a lot about Eric and his family. All the memories of Daddy abusing Mama rose to the surface. I told Eric that Daddy used to beat the hell out of Mama. It was something you didn't talk about in my small town in the 1970s. He had not understood the circumstances, and he apologized.

Three days later, I stepped away from the home I'd put a down payment on because it was going to be more expensive than I'd first thought. Instead of going through stages of grief with this loss over a period of weeks, I prayed and went within and experienced all the stages of house-grief in one night.

Whereas normally I cry and get overwhelmed, I handled each of those situations differently than I would have normally. There are karmic patterns that repeat, and my intuition allowed me to know the Universe was testing me. Yes, it was stressful. However, I didn't stay upset, I made different decisions, accepted things, and went with the flow. It made me understand I must change the way I think and handle situations. The key is to choose a different outcome in the lessons the Universe deals to us. *I feel like I played Monopoly, passed "Go," and collected $200.*

Chris' work schedule was heavy, and I wouldn't see him until the following weekend. One Sunday morning, after we had been involved for ten weeks, he arrived at my door. I hugged him. "We need to talk," he said. "I want to do it the right way." Chris said he would be working more, that I needed someone who would be with me more often. He'd received a Divinely guided message through his spiritual gift to not be a Dom anymore, and he thought I needed one. I told him, "No, you are wrong about that. The last time we were together I knew I wanted more than BDSM." *I want a loving relationship.*

He said, "I've had the same dream four days in a row. You don't belong to me."

"What do you mean?"

"You were with someone in the dream. It's the way you looked at him."

"Describe him."

"He is shorter than me, wider than me, and has more hair than me."

I couldn't breathe. I broke down. He'd seen my twin in the dreams. In tears, I asked, "Have you ever loved two people at the same time?"

"No."

"Do you remember me telling you I have a Twin Flame?"

"Yes."

"The affair wasn't just an affair. You know how I saw you through my third eye?"

"Yes."

"My twin's face morphed in front of me one morning at dawn." I gave a condensed version of the affair and told Chris how I'd realized that Erick was my Twin Flame.

I told Chris that we are both green-eyed. I see close up with my left eye and far away with the right. My twin sees the same but from opposite eyes. He mirrors me. My twin's heart beat in unison with mine when we were together. "I need to tell you, Chris, that when I fell in love with you, it wasn't because of your similarities. It's because of who you are."

"Are you seeing signs? Synchronicities?"

"Yes. I see his name everywhere. Part of his name is the name of a transportation company. I drove for two hours and saw three trucks with his name. An intimate kiss from him woke me up from a dead sleep on Christmas morning." I told him about the synchronicities I'd seen when I was leaving the lake the day I'd been there seeking clarity. Chris listened, and I continued. "When I went to the lake two evenings ago, my left ear buzzed when Spirit wanted my attention. I heard a noise, and the pitch in my ears changed. I turned to the noise, and a mother was pushing a wagon at the dock I visited and two boys jumped out of it. The boys were two-year-old *twins. I realized the synchronicity.* The affair was two years ago."

"Have you reached out to your twin?"

"Yes. Before you and I met." I sent him three messages from a burner phone. The last text I sent said, "If you don't want me to send any more texts, reply stop." Two minutes later, he responded, "Stop." He wasn't strong enough to leave his marriage. I went to the beach in January to separate myself from Erick's energy. When you and I had sex, Chris, I felt him. My twin and I have telepathy. I know you are my present. Erick is my past." Through tears, I said, "I need you to know I wouldn't have cheated on you. I would be faithful. I'm not a cheater. God brought you to me because I was stagnant. I couldn't move forward. You are a good man, kind and sweet. I already miss you." I hugged him one last time, and we said goodbye.

In ten minutes, my world shattered. I was in shock. Chris is the best version of a man I have known. *How could it be over?* I trusted him. I felt safe, as I hadn't in over a year. He told me on our first date that he would mark me, and he did. If there ever was "a good breakup," I experienced it with Chris. I would miss him and our playtime. I texted him my feelings—I wanted him to know how important he was to me.

After four weeks of being an emotional mess, I wrote him a letter with my deepest feelings. I hoped it would bring him back to me. After a few weeks of not getting a response, I gave up. I had to move forward with my life. Because of the raw loss I had been through with Erick, I understood that taking those first steps away from Chris would be difficult. Being heartbroken is horrible, but I still hurt over the loss of my twin. That feeling was amplified by the loss of my new love. I was devastated. *How will I get through abandonment and rejection again?* My faith was strong, and I continue to be challenged. *What else can go wrong?*

Chapter 9
Death and Acceptance

YouTube spiritual readers and psychic mediums gave me insight into my Twin Flame journey. I only listened to readers when they gave me true psychic hits. They have given me specific information that, without a true psychic gift, no one could know. I have seen portals form and orbs present in selected readers' readings. *They have a spiritual gift.*

I receive channeled songs more often than I used to. When it happens, I'm not listening to the radio or thinking about any particular song, but suddenly, words drop into my mind or a few notes can be heard, and I realize it's a song. I know the Divine or Erick's higher self is sending communication through the lyrics. The number of songs that have come to me since my awakening is close to 100. This form of psychic awareness is a spiritual gift.

After a month of not hearing from Chris and still being in love with Erick, I reached out to a psychic for a reading. A reading confirmed my deepest fears, which sent me into a tailspin. His journey was also difficult. In the reading, the psychic told me that it is likely Erick is in a controlling situation. I have felt there is something she holds over Erick's head. The reading backed up my thoughts. Mama and my step-dad's looming health issues took precedence over the full impact I felt from the reading.

On Monday morning, I was in a low place from the reading I'd received that past Friday. I sat at my work area in grief. I had prayed so much over the last few days for my twin and myself. In deep sadness, I felt what I can only describe as a warm/hot pulsing sensation in my solar plexus chakra, and the pulse moved up to my heart chakra. In a matter of moments, something Divine took the pain and sadness from me. It was supernatural, healing, and I felt the love of a higher power. I was thankful.

I told Mama what had happened—and that the Divine had taken away my heavy emotional burden. Although she didn't understand my spiritual path, she was happy that I believed in a higher power.

Mama's and my step-father's health had been declining over the last five months. The previous December, Mama suffered an intestinal obstruction that she never recovered from. Staying on top of her healthcare needs and running my business stretched me thin. Mama was in the hospital for a few days in April with a bout of colitis, which caused extreme weakness. She wasn't able to care for herself or my step-father, so she was staying with me. I slept on my recliner and gave her my bed. I became overwhelmed. *How will I be able to care for Mama while working?* It was a stressful time. I went into autopilot mode.

My step-father's health took a turn for the worse. Six hours after the pulsing sensation I'd had stopped, he passed away. I believe those healing pulses prepared me for my stepfather's death and what was to come. When I'd met him in 1987, I'd accepted him as a missing piece of my life. I loved him and accepted the fatherly love he gave in return. He loved Mama in ways that a child who had seen domestic violence can appreciate. I viewed him as my real father, and he provided me with stability for almost thirty-two years. He was not a perfect man, but I am grateful for him being the father I wanted and needed.

Preparing for the funeral, Mama and I discussed finding Brian. I'd been estranged from Brian for a few years, and Mama had had no recent contact with him. He is his own worst enemy, and he has made choices which led us to ask, "How can the same gene pool produce siblings that turn out so differently?" We couldn't reach him. Dread overcame me—I would have to contact Daddy to locate Brian.

It had been a few years since I'd walked away from the toxicity of Daddy and Brian. Both of them had pitted me against the other. They told lies. Daddy and Brian may be my blood relatives, but before my spiritual awakening, I'd removed their lower vibrational energy frequency from my life. I'd planned on never speaking with either of them again. I don't regret that decision, but now, I had to let Brian know about our step-father's passing.

Mama was near me, listening in, when I called Daddy. I was anxious about having to make the call. Daddy answered and said, "Hi, honey. How are you? It's so good to hear your voice." I told him with little emotion about my step-father's passing; that we were trying to reach Brian. He had gotten out of jail for drug trafficking and had been released because of the COVID-19 pandemic. He had several cell numbers, and Daddy verified the correct one. As Mama listened, she shot me a look. She'd decided suddenly that she didn't want Brian at the funeral. I asked Daddy not to tell Brian. He and I made small talk, and he told me how good it was to hear from me. I couldn't reciprocate the sentiment. I told him goodbye.

When the call ended, Mama said she was embarrassed by Brian and the trouble he was in—that's why she didn't want him at the funeral. Because of her declining health, I felt protective of her. I later found out that Daddy (or his sister) had told Brian anyway.

Two days after my step-father's death, Mama wasn't as alert as she usually was. She was weak, and it bothered me. As I was helping her back to bed, she slid down to the carpeted floor. I called for help from the local fire department. They picked Mama up and placed her on the bed. She was quiet most of the afternoon, becoming less conversational, more lethargic. "How are you feeling, Mama?" I knew in my gut something was wrong.

She was disoriented. She believed her deceased mother knew about my step-father's death.

"Why?" I asked.

"I have a date with Mother," Mama replied. *Granny died over ten years ago.*

I panicked. I knew of other spouses who have died a few days apart. I didn't want to alert anyone, but I was afraid of losing her. I had the bedroom door closed so Crystal wouldn't disturb Mama. She looked at the door and barked—as if someone was in my home. *Had Crystal sensed spirits or seen Angels coming to take Mama away?*

After speaking with a doctor, I called the ambulance to transport Mama to the hospital. "Mama," I said, "I need to send you to the Emergency Room. If I don't, I'm afraid you won't get to stay here with me." Stepping into the ambulance, I leaned down and hugged her as she lay on the gurney, afraid this would be the last time I would see her alive. "I love you, Mama," I said through tears. I was terrified.

I took a list of Mama's medicines to the hospital. With the COVID-19 pandemic, the emergency room wouldn't let me in to see her. I left, knowing I might never see her again. I was shell shocked. I drove. *How could I lose both parents within two days?*

Close to home, I heard "Nothing Compares to You" on the radio. It took me back to Erick and me in bed one morning, sharing intimate thoughts. He pulled my short hair back and said, "You could shave your head like Sinead," implying I would look good bald.

"No," I said, "I won't," and laughed. Snapping back into reality, I realized I had driven into a parking lot. All I could do was move my gearshift into park.

Turning the radio off, I went into hysterics. Once I started screaming, I couldn't stop. "God, help me! Erick, help me! God help me! Erick, help me!" I thrashed my head back and forth against the seat. After I stopped, I sat there in shock. I couldn't move. In the depth of my despair, I felt coolness around my shoulders. I knew Angels were wrapping their loving arms around me. I sat in the dark, deserted parking lot alone. I begged God, "Please don't take Mama from me. I'm not ready to give her up." I lost track of time. I heard the song "Diamond Girl," by Seals and Crofts clairaudiently. It was a song I may have heard a few times in my life but never really listened to.

After a while, I settled and noticed my surroundings. I drove to my apartment. I parked and sat in my car. My limbs felt like dead weight. Something made me look up the lyrics for "Diamond Girl" on my cell phone. There was a reference to what Erick had called me, a "shining star," and I knew that a part of Erick was within me. I realized Erick had felt my energy shift—or his higher self had sent me the song to soothe me.

The next morning, I received a call. I was overjoyed to hear Mama's voice. "You did good," she said, meaning that she had arrived at the hospital at the right time. I knew God had answered my prayer. He didn't take Mama, and I felt grateful. Mama's health began improving, but she wouldn't be able to live alone anymore. My one-bedroom apartment was too small for us.

I reconnected with a childhood friend, Jenna, who is a realtor. She showed me multiple listings and helped me find our new home. It was the perfect place for Mama and me. She would have a walk-in shower and covered patio to enjoy. It allowed me to have a large home office. I put an offer on it and held my breath that it would be accepted. Opening up about spirituality, I found that Jenna and I shared similar views. We talked more and bounced beliefs and ideas back and forth. My offer was accepted, and I closed on my new home in June—I was excited that Mama could live with me after her hospital stay.

Hospital physicians suggested a rehabilitative stay at a nursing home. Samantha and I delivered Mama to the nursing home in late May. Mama had such a positive attitude about going to the nursing home and getting her strength back to begin the next phase of her life. Two days later, Mama fell and hit her head, and her injuries needed to be evaluated at the hospital. The bruising over her left eye surprised me. It covered her left eye, but there was deep bruising above her eyebrow that extended to the left side of her nose. Remembering the facial bruising that had happened with my fall, I knew the site would swell, expand, and darken in the coming days. She was less alert, and I enacted her medical power of attorney, which enabled me to make necessary decisions.

Mama fell again in the hospital. This time it was worse. She'd gotten out of bed with no one knowing. I went to the hospital and was shocked—the bruising on her left eye area was compounded by the second fall. Between her healthcare supervision, packing up both her home and my apartment, and continuing to run my business, I was worried. *Can I take care of everything?*

Over the next few days, Mama's health and cognitive behavior declined. She grew weaker each day, but multiple doctors could not give a definitive diagnosis. They were at a loss for what was wrong. I allowed a spinal tap. They wheeled her away for the test, and I sat in her room and prayed for a diagnosis so they could save my sweet Mama. I felt that my breakup with Chris had happened because I had to be with Mama during this time.

The spinal tap test was inconclusive, and I was distraught at the possibility of losing Mama. The daily hospital visits were heart-wrenching because there were no answers for why she wasn't improving. Mama slept most of the day.

I had reached my limit. I couldn't take any more. I pushed myself and was exhausted. Visitation at the hospital became about me having quiet time to allow my brain to slow down and my body to rest. I prayed. *I realize how delicate life is.*

After Mama's fall, Brian and I exchanged words through text. In honoring Mama's request of not sharing information with him, I kept the seriousness of her illness from him. She didn't need his shit show around her. After Mama's two falls, he wanted to know about her health. "She can't talk to you," I said. "Her condition is delicate. She is in a rehab nursing home. She has already said that she doesn't want to see you because of the trouble you are in. I can't be around you because of my work. I can't have any doubt upon me." *Being associated with him could cause me to lose my job.* "She will be okay."

He said, "I wasn't going to tell her about my arrest."

I said, "She had the right to know. You are her son, and she loves you, but she cannot be upset right now. She said she would be upset if she saw or talked to you." *All true.*

He left me an angry voicemail and spewed anger at me. "You turned Mama against me."

I texted him and said, "I am blocking you from future contact with me. I didn't turn Mama against you. Your own actions over the last 35 years did. You have played the victim so many times I've lost count, stretched the truth into your own delusional version of the truth, which is lies. So many people have helped you over the years, yet you continue to screw up your own life and take financially and emotionally from people that loved you at one time. Mama has told me she doesn't want you in her life, and I will abide by her wishes. Do not contact me ever again. I am done with you and the toxicity you bring whenever you are around. Goodbye."

Each day in the hospital Mama became weaker, unable to sip liquids on her own or to swallow medicine. The situation was dire. Mama has always been plus-size, and she had lost weight. Her face was sunken. Neurology was offering the possibility of dementia, but I didn't want to accept that.

I allowed a feeding tube. I told my exhausted Mama that she wasn't getting nutrition and needed to have the tube inserted. The nurses asked me to step outside her room while they did the procedure. I heard Mama moan and knew she was in pain.

Two mornings later, I received a call from her. "Come and get me," she said. "This hospital is starving me." A physician said Mama was delusional. I made all the necessary decisions and started a conservatorship, something I never thought I would have to do.

The next morning, Mama called. "I'm better," she said. "You can come get me."

"You aren't well enough to come home," I told her. I drove to the hospital to check on her. I walked into her room and couldn't believe my eyes. Mama was sitting in a chair, smiling, and talking to me! A doctor had changed one medication overnight. The nurses removed her feeding tube, and she'd started eating and drinking without help. I knew beyond a doubt—Mama's recovery was a miracle!

While I was sitting at a red light outside the hospital, "You Make Me Feel Brand New" came on the radio. The lyrics made me think of Erick. As I was waiting, a car caught my eye—*was it Erick's*? The driver looked back at me in his rear-view mirror. I had to know if it was Erick—and followed the vehicle. He turned into his driveway—it was him! The Divine had brought us together in that moment. Ironically, it was a year after we'd gone to court. As I drove away, I heard "Diamond Girl" and "Miracles" played on the radio consecutively.

Mama's quick improvement allowed her to return to the nursing home, and she worked hard to regain her strength. Without worrying as much about Mama's health, I could move forward. I packed up her home and my apartment. I felt such an accomplishment being single and closing on our new home, which would soon be conducive to Mama's needs. Close family and friends helped me finish everything I couldn't do alone, and I will always be grateful. Mama regained her strength and prepared to leave rehab and move in with me. Knowing Mama would come home in a few short days, I took a quick trip alone to the mountains. Erick stayed on my mind. I thought of him while driving. As I approached a transport truck with his name emblazoned on the side, "Green-Eyed Lady" played on the radio. *Another synchronicity from the Universe.*

Connecting with nature, I walked a trail and listened to the rushing water. That night, I escaped and numbed out. I was in the pain body again. I couldn't escape it. I remembered the morning I had watched Erick curled up on the shower floor. Tears of sadness mixed with shower droplets fell on me as I lay on the hotel shower floor. That night, I dreamed of him: There were two conferences inside one room. Erick and I were both in attendance. He walked behind me, put his hands on the top of my chair, leaned down, and heard his voice whisper in my ear, "It is what it is." After that, he and Karen were on top of a two-story garage, arguing. She saw me. I woke up wishing I could stay in the mountains, but it was time to return home. Mama was coming to her new home, moving in with me, the next day.

After two months of difficulties, it was time to pick Mama up from the nursing home. We hired caregivers to aid her because I needed to run my business. She invited family and friends into our new home. It took multiple efforts to pull everything together, and Mama's laughter made everything worth it. Watching her use a walker seemed like a miracle—I'd seen her near death just a few short weeks ago.

Mama had been with me four nights when I awoke to hear her coughing. It concerned me, given that COVID-19 was prevalent. She said, "It's nothing," but she also had a fever. Her doctor's office recommended she return to the hospital to be checked for COVID-19. She refused. "If you get worse, you will have to go to the hospital, Mama," I told her.

Mama took comfort medicine, and her fever lowered. She improved, but she went to bed early that night.

On Thursday morning, concerned, the caregiver asked me to come downstairs. I found Mama up, using her walker. But she was confused and disoriented. When I checked her temperature, it was almost 103. She jabbed me with a lancet while she was trying to check her blood-sugar level. "I'm calling the ambulance," I told her. The first responders arrived, and Mama refused to go to the hospital. I realized she didn't want to go because she was afraid of not returning home. After some coaxing, she went by ambulance to hospital. The nurses called. Mama had a bad UTI.

The next morning, the hospital called. Mama was COVID-19 positive. I developed a cough. After being tested, I returned home and slept. Over the next few days, my cough worsened, my fever increased to between 102 – 104, and my pulse ox was 92 to 93. A rash developed on my face and torso that resembled poison ivy, and I had nausea with a persistent headache. I didn't need test results to know I was COVID-19 positive. I had to manage Mama's health from my bed.

Mama's health declined, and they moved her to CCU because the nurses didn't like the way she looked. I talked with God and prayed. Not only worried about Mama's health, I also had mine to think about. *Will I end up in the hospital, too?* The nausea was terrible. I lost ten pounds in a few days. I was fatigued and weak. I became resigned. Talking with God, I accepted my fate but asked that if it was not my time to go, to allow me to live. Also, I asked that Archangel Raphael, who is in charge of physical healing, come into my presence and heal me.

It was all I could do to take care of myself and stay involved in Mama's medical decisions. The continued calls with the hospital showed Mama wasn't doing well. Sometimes she was lucid; other times she was out of her head. A hospitalist called requesting a transcatheter cardiac procedure. Knowing Mama only had hypertension without other heart disease, I declined the procedure. The cardiologist then said, "I don't think it's her heart," and I thought, *Why did this even get suggested to me?* Mama had made her wishes known to me when my step-father had died. I accepted it was only a matter of time until God called Mama home.

I told God, "I'm ready. Bring Mama home. I don't want her to suffer anymore." The next morning, I received a call that Mama was pulling at her BiPap machine. Knowing Mama was tired, I told the staff to make her comfortable. I knew she would want that. Later that afternoon, her health took a rapid decline, and she passed away that afternoon. God answered my prayer—Mama was no longer suffering.

I felt the explosion of deep soul pain in losing her. My mama was gone. I sobbed. Reality set in—I was alone. I had no immediate family—I'd removed Daddy and Brian from my life. I was an orphan. I found my grandmother's strength and didn't lie in my grief.

I knew I had to tell Brian. I unblocked his number from my phone. The hospital wouldn't have let Brian in to see Mama because she was COVID-19 positive. I should have told him as her health worsened, but with me being sick, I didn't reach out to him. *I didn't think she would die.* Our strained situation was only going to get worse. I took a deep breath to figure out the words to text.

I started texting:

Mama's suffered so much with health issues since December. She's been in and out of the hospital and nursing rehab since April 30. She came to live with me on 7/10. I continued to ask her if she wanted me to contact you and her answer was always no. On 7/16, she went to the ER and had a UTI. On 7/17, the hospital called, and she had Covid. Her health continued to go down. The hospital called today. Her health took a rapid decline, and she passed away peacefully about an hour ago. The funeral will be delayed as I am recovering from Covid. I will send you information about the funeral when I have it.

After receiving clearance from a doctor, I planned Mama's Celebration of Life Service and notified Brian. She hadn't wanted a traditional funeral. She had written her memories down a couple of years before and had wanted someone to read them at visitation. Although I have an aversion to public speaking (a trait Erick shared), I looked for Mama's memories. I'd moved into my home, but some things remained unpacked. No matter where I looked, I couldn't find the information. I tore my house apart looking for her memories and gave the situation over to God. I moved forward and wrote my speech. I accepted that I wouldn't find Mama's memories, and suddenly their location dropped into my mind. I couldn't believe it! I found the words she had written. *The Divine gave me the answer.*

It was time to see Mama's body before the public visitation. She lay in a wooden casket that was draped in a multi-colored quilt my great-grandmother had made years ago. It was the same one that had been used for Granny's funeral. While I was looking at Mama's corpse, I realized, *It's her empty shell—her radiant smile and contagious laughter are gone.* Sitting alone and waiting for visitation, I felt empty. I dreaded Brian and I being alone during the family viewing. For unknown reasons, he didn't come in during this time. As I sat there meditating, my second-cousin Sadie arrived and comforted me.

Sadie's mother was Granny's sister, so while Sadie is Mama's cousin, they were more like sisters. She is in some of my earliest memories and has always been warm and kind. As I became an adult and was busier, I lost touch with her—for twenty years. Sadie had supported me through Mama's illness and our move, and had become my rock; someone I could always count on. Sadie invited me to be an active part of future family functions. Her sons treat me like a sister. With her in my life and the love she and her family give me, I don't feel alone. I am grateful.

Brian and I didn't speak at the visitation. We ignored each other—no eye contact. It was awkward. He spent a large amount of time outside the funeral home. I believe he was using drugs in the parking lot. My son Kurt hadn't spoken to me in fifteen months and didn't respond when I told him his grandmother had passed away. He punished me by not being a pallbearer. It hurt me because he didn't respect Mama enough to do this last kindness for her. Holding a grudge is something he learned from me, and I acknowledge that.

Two synchronicities happened with Mama's death. When I received her death certificate, I saw that someone named Eric was the embalmer, which made me shake my head—that's more than mere coincidence. Walking through the funeral home before her service, I saw older photos from historical time periods hanging on the walls. I felt drawn to one and walked over to look at it. Beneath the photo were the names of the people in it. One name listed was Erik. I missed Erick. He always had the right words to calm me.

As I prepared the last moments before walking to the podium, I closed my eyes and prayed to God to help me deliver the speech in a way to honor Mama without becoming emotional. I was nervous. I approached the podium and right before I opened my mouth, I felt Erick's energy come to me. It gave me strength. It was as if he knew at that moment I needed him. *Was it his 3D self thinking about me, or was it his higher self?* In the end, I honored Mama and hoped she was proud of me.

As I approached the graveyard, I heard "Diamond Girl" on the radio—the same song that had come to me the night I thought I was losing Mama. *Synchronicity.* Brian walked over to me and made the effort to give me a simple hug. My guard was up.

Brian said, "I know you hate me."

"No, I don't."

He walked away.

I didn't hate him, but I would keep my distance from him because he had been involved in drug trafficking. On my way home, I heard "Love Will Turn You Around." Mama and I both loved that song, and I hadn't heard it in twenty-five years. That was a nod from the Divine, and I smiled. *Mama is with me in spirit.*

The last few months had taken their toll on me, but I knew Mama wouldn't want me to mourn her. I am not angry or bitter about losing Mama. I am accepting. My new life without Mama would be different; uncharted. I became executrix of the estate and had a new set of challenges because Mama had cut Brian and a step-sister from the will. In the will, she stated that they had received their portion of inheritance during her lifetime. Brian told Sadie he wasn't angry, but I knew damn well he was pissed off.

In the coming days, I had to start my new role as executrix. All I can say is God is with me and His Angels continue to guide, direct, and protect me. I feel the Divine around me at all times. If you had told me six months before I would trust in an unknown, higher power, I wouldn't have thought it possible. Yet, it is. Every part of me knows I have become more spiritual than I ever thought possible. I see beyond 3D illusion. I have spiritual gifts, and I feel close to God without religion.

My heart misses Erick. We are two halves of the same soul, and I'm incomplete without him. I realized the Twin Flame journey is about me and my healing, not just about Erick. I want to know what my spiritual mission is. I'm not sure what will happen next. Things are revealed when the timing is right. For now, I move forward and embrace life.

Chapter 10
Forgiving and Surrendering

Two weeks after Mama's death, as my spirituality grew deeper, I felt led to forgive anyone I'd held hard feelings for in my heart. My list began with twelve people and it grew to thirty-four. The wounds I had were painful. I realized true forgiveness was going to take longer than I'd thought.

Some people were easier to forgive. Erick would be last—the deep wounds he'd caused me would be the last ones I released. I heard the song "Heart of the Matter" by Don Henley repeatedly. I felt Spirit prod me to forgive Erick more quickly than I'd intended. During this time, YouTube suggested a video about concentration camp survivors. This subject both fascinates and horrifies me—but I watched it. The video told the story of Eva Mozes Kor and her twin, who suffered experiments created by Dr. Josef Mengele during World War II. They took her to Auschwitz, her family was separated, and she underwent horrific experiments. She had a life-threatening fever, but she still forgave Mengele. Instead of hating this man and others whose actions had led to the loss of her family members, she forgave them. She didn't allow hate to remain in her heart.

I sat with my feelings. They felt so minor: all my perceived injustices were insignificant compared to hers. I allowed what I saw and heard to digest, and it struck a nerve within me. *If Eva can heal and forgive, how can I not?* It was a powerful moment. I was supposed to see that video. At that moment, I knew I had to forgive everyone. I decided to text Erick on a cell phone I wasn't using.

My closest friends knew I was in a period of forgiveness, but only Melissa knew and supported my decision to send Erick a text because I was being guided to do it. Erick may not be with me, but I knew he didn't want to hurt anyone. In fact, he is empathic and feels terrible when he sees an injustice. I wanted him to know I don't hate him. I dug deep to not be in ego or pride when selecting words I felt he might need to hear:

> *Told that I need to forgive. "Heart of the Matter" was engrained in my mind. Watched a video about a concentration twin survivor and the experiments done to them. Turned into a message of forgiveness. You were the last one on my list. I was pushed to act more quickly by a higher power. People hurt each other. It happens to everyone and is what we do. Intentionally, unintentionally, regretfully or not. We can heal and forgive. When one forgives, two are healed. There's no love without forgiveness, and there's no forgiveness without love. We can't heal until we forgive. Forgiveness doesn't make you weak, but it is a gift and sets you free. It frees up your power, heals your body, mind, soul, and spirit. You'll never know how strong your heart is until you know how to forgive who broke it. SOS 34.*[6]

---

[6] "I Have Found the One My Soul Loves" – Song of Solomon 3:4 KJV

I asked Melissa, "Do you think it's time for me to send the message?" She encouraged me. She rode with me to ensure Erick was at work so there was no risk of my text message being intercepted. On our way to his office, we saw a murder of crows. We both smiled, knowing the crow is a spirit animal for me. We saw a license plate with 1111, the Twin Flame number. We both said, "That's a synchronicity." I held my breath and hit send. I knew I'd done the right thing. I felt better. I had no expectations.

After I sent the message to Erick, I realized I'd held grudges against others for insignificant things. Yes, some hurt more deeply. I looked at it from both sides. For the first time, I allowed myself to have forgiveness in my heart.

The hardest situation took a month to work through: forgiving Daddy. Fathers are supposed to be a daughter's safety net. Mine was not. Fathers are supposed to be loving towards their wives, and Daddy was the polar opposite of that. Even though my parents had divorced forty years ago, I still remember Mama's cries when Daddy abused her when he was drunk. I retrieved painful repressed memories and tried to move past them. The images are still vivid. One of the worst things happened was on the day they inaugurated Ronald Reagan in 1981. Brian was fourteen; I was eleven. Without permission, Brian took Daddy's new car for a joyride in the snow. He totaled it and awaited Daddy coming home. Brian begged me to call my grandpa and have him pick him up; he was terrified of Daddy's rage.

I made the call to my grandpa and expressed my concern. "It will be okay," he said. I hoped it would. I covered my ears in my bedroom as Brian screamed. Each lash from Daddy's belt caused me to push my fingers into my ears and grit my teeth, hoping it would block out every sound. But it didn't work. The beating left belt marks over Brian's back and legs. I don't know how I escaped Daddy's wrath, but to this day I am grateful that he never whipped me.

Daddy had a long list of infractions. Every injustice that happened within my immediate family that shaped me had to be relived in my mind. I walked into each painful moment and allowed myself to no longer live in fear. Forgiving Daddy was an emotional release necessary for me to have peace in my life.

The last thing was checked off the list. I felt grateful to God that I had forgiven Daddy. Even though I forgave him, I never needed to see or speak to him ever again. You don't need to invite toxicity back in once you rid yourself of it. I'd held grudges for years and had only hurt myself. God and spirituality allowed me to let go of what was holding me back from healing wounds. I am grateful for the powerful lesson that came through His grace and love.

Over the next couple of months, I felt joy and happiness again—with occasional dips of sadness. I looked for signs, synchronicities, and healing for my soul contract. Even though I had work to do, I opened myself up to live life. I remembered Erick's words: "We can't depend on others for our own happiness."

In my period of forgiveness, I decided I needed to resolve the karma between Greg and me. How do you apologize to someone when everything you did over five months could be counted amongst your worst behaviors ever? *I destroyed his life.* I knew he had been seeing someone and hoped he was happy. He deserved that. I exhaled as I began drafting a text:

> *I wanted to tell you I've been thinking about many things and have been working on myself. Greg, I want to apologize to you for my actions and the way I ended our marriage, the lies I told, and for the damage and hurt I caused you. There is nothing I can do other than to say that. I AM sorry for all that happened. The lies are something I regret and only made the situation worse. I am glad you have found someone to love you like I couldn't, I mean that. I wish you and her happiness.*

He didn't reply. I deserved that. Later, Roman told me Greg was remarrying. I smiled. *He is getting his happy ending.*

On New Year's Eve, I went to my bank. I wanted to get take-home meals for the holiday weekend. Driving by a cafe restaurant in the mid-afternoon, I felt drawn to stop there. While at the bank, I saw silver spots and flecks in the sky. I smiled, knowing they were from my Angel team. It reminded me that I am guided, directed, and protected, and inspired me to text Melissa. "The Angels are all up in my business today," I typed.

After I left the bank, I went to the restaurant. I saw a truck identical to Erick's. As I sat in my vehicle, I was excited and anxious. *Is he alone? I won't let it stop me if she is with him.* I was wearing my light green COVID-19 mask. When I walked inside, I became hyper-aware of every face I looked at. I didn't see him at first. When I saw the back of his head, my heart felt as if it was going to burst. *You wore that same green sweater two years ago, and it still looks good on you. You really need tighter jeans.*

A few people stood between us. They were indecisive with their order. They offered to let me go in front of them. I walked to his left as he ordered. Erick had a list in his hand. My appearance had changed since we'd last seen each other. I didn't know if he saw me, but I placed my order. Unsure if he heard my voice, I ordered a favorite food of ours, mashed potatoes. He moved behind me, then to the counter to pick up his food. If he had seen me, he said nothing.

Erick walked to the front to pay the cashier. There was a lady standing between us. He waited in line and talked to her. Erick looked past her and glanced into my eyes, and did a double take. *Did he hear me but, because my hair is longer and darker, didn't think it was me? Maybe he feels my energy.* He knew me even with my mask on. Our eyes locked—it was as if it was just the two of us there. He couldn't quit looking at me, nor I at him. At the cash register, he turned sideways towards me, smiling through his mask, and seemed to wait for me after he paid for his food. Then he exited and walked towards his truck. I walked to the cashier to pay for my meals. *Can she go any slower?!* As I walked towards his truck, I saw he had rolled his window down and sat inside. He was waiting for me. I couldn't decide how close to get to him, and allowed three feet between us.

Erick said, "You look good. Oh my God, you look good." *I should've washed my hair.*

Our eyes met. I said, "You do, too."

"I saw your little eyes look up at me."

"Have you seen me in town?" I asked.

"No. But I have been looking for you. How are you?"

"A lot has happened," I said. "Mama brought COVID home from the nursing home, and we both got it. She passed away. I made it. Did you know she had died?"

"No," he said. "I'm so sorry." *He is.*

"I'm okay."

I believe Erick was glad to see me. He was at ease and very warm. My ego stepped in. I said court was hard on all of us. He looked at me. I couldn't stop the words "Karen borderline stalked me. She is crazy!"

He said nothing.

"Do you feel me?" I asked. "Because I feel you." *Telepathically, sexually.* I don't think he knew what to say. He wouldn't look me in the eye. It was as if he knew what I meant. My thoughts weren't contained. "Do you still love me?"

He was facing forward in his truck and wouldn't look at me but said, "No."

I made you uncomfortable by asking, and you turned away. "Look me in the eye and tell me that," I said. *Damn it, look at me.*

There was a moment of hesitation. He breathed in, turned toward me, and, looking at me, said, "I don't love you." *Please God, don't let me cry.*

I asked, "Do you know how many tears I've cried?" Realizing I didn't want him to feel guilty with my words, I said, "I'm not trying to make you feel bad." Wanting to contain my deep feelings, I said, "It doesn't really matter, I'm just saying."

Erick said nothing. *Let me disappear.*

I wanted to run. I knew I needed to exit gracefully. I said, "You could have given me closure."

"I give you closure," he said gently.

"That's what I needed to hear," I said. I turned away and walked to my car. I saw his truck stop behind me. He had stopped for a vehicle in front of him. We exited the parking lot in opposite directions.

I was empty. In shock. As I drove home, my emotions were rising to the surface. When I got home, I started feeling. Tears were falling. It was New Year's Eve. I sat on the cold wooden floor of my bedroom closet with a thick blanket, numbing out. The images and words replayed in my head. *Why have I held on? Did I imagine him caring for me?* I was trying to wrap my head around what had unfolded. I wanted to understand everything that had happened between us. I felt he never deserved me or my love, which made me cry more.

That night, I lay in my infinite sadness. Another dark night of the soul was upon me. Though I had forgiven Erick three months ago, I was triggered heavily in response to his rejection. Through swollen eyes and little tears remaining, I said aloud, "You abandoned me. You betrayed me. You chose her. You rejected me. You broke me!" Every core wound ripped through my heart. The pain of losing Mama didn't compare. I prayed: "God help me to change. Stop my vicious cycle of not moving forward. Help me quit feeling this pain body I have lived in for almost two years. I need to move forward. I want to move forward."

I reflected. After a couple of weeks, I told myself, "It's a new year. I will do things differently. But my unconditional love for Erick will remain. My clairsentience gift made me feel, *when he said he didn't love me, he was lying—he'd hesitated before looking me in the eye.* But, he had made his choice to stay nearly two years ago. I allowed myself to mourn. I prayed for a high-level soulmate to be brought into my life. God gave me an enormous heart to love no matter what traumatic scars were deep inside me.

Part of my Twin Flame journey has been realizing that we, as a spiritual collective, are supposed to love others unconditionally. The only time I had felt this before Erick was through the birth of my children. Once I accepted this, I took baby steps. I opened my heart chakra, and I knew it wouldn't be a simple process.

There are several stages in a Twin Flame connection. Ones I consider part of my journey are:

1. recognizing your twin,
2. awakening spiritually,
3. being attracted magnetically,
4. being tested,
5. experiencing a dark night of the soul,
6. running/chasing,
7. being separated,
8. surrendering the connection, and
9. releasing attachment to outcome.

I've surrendered this and have made it through eight stages. I decided I wanted—no, needed—the ninth stage. I would be open and no longer resist the Divine.

Chapter 11

Transforming and Dreaming

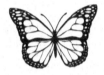

It was mid-January, and I settled back into my quiet life. Charles, the maintenance guy from the apartments, invited me to a karaoke bar. Wanting a male friend in my life, I agreed to go. Although I'm not a singer, Charles encouraged me to get on stage. I don't have a "bucket list," but I wanted to sing karaoke just so I could say I'd done it. Sitting at the pub-style table, I chose two of the songs I'd heard clairaudiently, "Miracles" and "Diamond Girl." To keep my anxiety at bay, I drank rum and Coke. As I approached the microphone, I asked myself, *"Are you really going to do this?"* My mouth opened, and I sang both songs to a small crowd. I finished, knowing I'd done something outside my comfort zone. *At least they didn't boo me off the stage.*

After Mama's death, most weekends included a visit to my cousin Sadie's home. I knew Sadie loved me—she offered me stability and was my surrogate mother. I felt blessed to not feel like an orphan. I can't imagine where I'd be without her. Her sons and their families welcomed Roman and me with open arms into a loving and safe atmosphere.

I loved the peaceful mornings when I walked Crystal. It felt like I was getting my footing back after seeing Erick. On a Sunday morning in mid-January, I received a text from Chris. He had exited my life almost nine months earlier, and I realized how much I missed him. He wanted to come and see me. My doorbell rang, and I greeted him with a hug. We talked about our lives since last seeing one another. I didn't ask him why he'd reappeared.

I told Chris I was going to have a Mommy Makeover procedure in April, which included breast reduction, abdominoplasty, and liposuction. *My middle section needs this.*

"Why?" he asked.

"I'm tired of back, neck, and shoulder pain and numbness."

"You look fine the way you are," he said.

His reassurance is one reason I had fallen in love with him. He wanted to see my new place, and I showed him my new spiritual closet. There is a small desk and huge bean bag chair against the wall, and many of my tarot and oracle cards hang on a shoe organizer on the door. While we stood in the closet, we both saw an energy shift—it looked like vertical waves on the straight wall. It was unexplainable, like a break in the 3D matrix.

"What do you think it means?" Chris asked.

"I don't know," I said. I was sorry to see him go but happy for the time we had shared. Hugging him, I kissed him on the side of his cheek and lips. If Chris was being brought back into my life, I would accept him. Over the next week, we exchanged many texts, which made me remember why I had missed him. I'd told him I wanted to feel more confident handling my handgun, and he asked if I would like to go on a date to a shooting range.

At the shooting range, I saw Chris could take someone out—he was an excellent shot. After he helped me out with my handgun, we had dinner at an Italian Restaurant in our city. We talked and reminisced. "Why did you contact me?" I asked.

"Because I still love and miss you."

That made me happy. *But would we stay in each other's lives?* I didn't see Chris for a few weeks after that. Chris and I are both Virgos. We go within when things are heavy on our hearts and we are deep in our heads. A close friend of his had contracted COVID-19 and had died. As a result of a big winter storm, he had to work long hours at his commercial properties. I gave him his space. He came by one Sunday morning. We sat down and caught up. He had helped the family of his friend through their loss. My heart felt heavy for him, as I know the deep loss of a COVID-19-related death.

"Let's talk about our relationship," I said. Spirit had given Chris answers through his visions. They had shown "her" to Chris. He described her, and I told him I hope he finds her this lifetime. Through his vision, he also saw that I would find love in my life. "You will remarry and be happy," he said.

By now, the tears that were dammed up behind my eyes fell down my cheeks. "I asked God to not let me cry," I said. "But I just can't be strong enough." I let him see me with my imperfections.

The wall between us was removed. "Who do you see me marrying?" I asked. "If I show you a photo of someone, can you tell me if it was the same person you saw in your vision?"

"Sure."

I pulled out my cell phone and showed him Erick's photo. "Is this who you saw?"

He said, "He is wider in the picture but very similar." *I found the photo last year on the Internet. Erick has gained some weight and is heavier than when we were together.*

I divulged more about Erick that I hadn't shared with him earlier, the previous April. As I told Chris about Erick, the man I love unconditionally, and what transpired between us, my tears flowed. Chris never interrupted me; he just listened. I made no apology, just allowed the emotions to be released. I put my hand on his chest. The tone of my voice varied as I sobbed. I told him how much he means to me, that I will always love him unconditionally, and he will stay in my heart. He said I am a good woman. It seemed difficult for him to not lose his composure. We said goodbye for a second time. I hugged him before he walked out of my life again.

How I handle an ending to a romantic situation when it's not my choice can send me into a spiral. I love deeply. It's how God wired me. For many years, I wouldn't allow my feelings and heart to be transparent, but my awakening transformed me into a better version of myself. It allowed me to be vulnerable. Growing up, I felt it was a weakness to cry in front of others.

After Chris left, I prayed to be helped through another loss. Within thirty minutes of him leaving and praying for God to help me again through another disappointment in love, my tears stopped. I looked around my living room and felt the Divine lift the situation from me. I sent Chris a text: "Thank you for giving me closure. It was what I needed. I felt abandoned and rejected, but now I don't. It's part of my healing."

I was feeling low, but I had something to look forward to—in just two weeks I was going to Panama City Beach with Samantha and Roman to hang out in a condo on the beach. While we were there, I spent most of the time relaxing as the waves crashed against the shoreline. *Ahhh...the sound of the ocean waves crashing took my ear buzzing away.* The weather was nice, and I relaxed. We got sunburned on St. Patrick's Day.

That week I dreamed about Erick and Daddy, from whom I am still estranged. The dreams were lucid and woke me up. The first dream involved me walking into a seventies-style home with a partition opening between a living room and kitchen. Through a cutout between rooms, I saw Erick walking toward me with a huge smile on his face. I felt guarded. He reached inside his right shirt pocket and pulled a handmade steel-wire ring out and wanted to hold my right hand. He placed the ring on my right ring finger. Tears of joy filled both of our eyes. Erick expressed his love to me. Someone in the kitchen said, "Finally!"

In another dream, Daddy came into my bedroom. He wanted to speak with me. It was as if a dream was within that dream, like I had forgotten him. I walked outside and discovered Brian had driven Daddy to my home. I didn't care if I spoke to him or not. *I've never dreamed of Daddy.* I woke up knowing his time on earth was ending. He was going to die. I was being given a last opportunity to see and talk to him if I wanted. I shared this with close friends and decided I didn't need to see him. I felt at peace with my decision.

Ten days after I had the dream, Sadie called, telling me Daddy had died. My dream had been a premonition. Many thoughts and memories came to me, but for twenty-four hours, I remained unemotional. I called Brian to get the funeral arrangements, but I never received a return call. I became anxious—I had to decide whether I would attend the funeral.

Daddy's death sunk in. I became emotional. Many memories surfaced. I remembered his physical and emotional abuse of Mama and Brian again; how he'd come home drunk so many times. I'd been relieved when he'd get home after I was in bed. After his death, my fear of him remained. Visualizing my terrified younger self in a traumatic moment, my current self went to that little girl. I took her hand and walked her away from the violence. I told her she's loved, that none of what happened was her fault. Many daughters love their fathers, but mine caused many of my childhood emotional wounds. Although I forgave him last year, the memories remain. I numbed out while grieving in my own way.

I was mad as hell when I read Daddy's obituary in black and white: "He will be remembered as a loving husband and father." Disgust, dizziness, and nausea overcame me. My thoughts transitioned to attending his funeral. *It's expected… What will people think if I don't go?* It was overwhelming. I was afraid of seeing Brian. I reached out to Chris. "Will you go with me?" I asked. "I don't think I can go alone." *I want him there in case Brian causes trouble.* Knowing we will always have a loving and respectful bond, I needed a piece of his inner strength. Even though his schedule was busy, he agreed to go with me.

My Aunt Lauren, whom I love, gave me the best insight:

Considering the circumstances of your relationship over the last fifty years, I wouldn't go to the funeral or gravesite. Why drag up hurtful memories? Do what's best for you. That's what he did. You may be even more upset if you hear his eulogy and it sugarcoats his life, which it will. That's standard procedure. I'll support you whatever you decide to do. Your feelings are what's important. Only you can decide. Don't let anyone convince you to go if you don't want to.

Close family and friends gave me advice and permission to honor my feelings. After two days, I heard my inner voice. *What do you want to do?* In that defining moment, I made my decision. A childhood friend who had lived in the house beside us when Daddy abused Mama had graciously offered to go with me to the funeral home, but I declined. I wouldn't go to the visitation, funeral, or burial. My higher self gave me inner peace, which was needed. I texted the people closest to me:

When I read his obituary yesterday, I was mad as hell and felt as if I was going to vomit. I witnessed horrors no small child should have seen. Hearing my inner voice, I realized I was going to go out of a sense of obligation. Last year, I made peace with him. In a dream, I decided if I wanted to talk to him one last time. I don't have to go. I don't hate

Daddy, but my stepdad was my father. Mama could've turned me against Daddy, but she didn't. I am choosing myself and my feelings over what's expected. That is part of this lesson. Other people put emotions on us. I have put others ahead of myself most of my life, and this time, I honor myself and my feelings. Daddy's corpse is just that. Not him. Looking at him in a casket or listening to the eulogy will injure me more, and I can't do it. People won't understand, but I am at peace with my decision, which will lead to healing.

I thanked Chris for being willing to go with me and shared my text with him. He was well aware of how Daddy's death could have sent me into a spiral. He brought me strength I sometimes lack. I texted him, "There was nothing I could receive by attending the funeral."

He replied, "You know you can always draw strength from me when you need it! I respect and congratulate you on your decision and do hope to see you continue to grow! I will always leave a special channel for you to draw from."

The day of the funeral came. I worked. *I'm resolved and glad it's over.*

Charles had supported my decision to not attend Daddy's funeral. His friendship mattered to me, and I kept him in the friends-only zone. I had my first post-COVID-19 work conference coming to Texas. Because I didn't want to travel alone, I asked Charles if he would go with me. He was happy to take off a few days from work.

We hit a few of the local restaurants with bars. The locals were friendly, and the food was delicious. I loved one of the bars inside the fancy hotel, as there are many plants, trees, and flowers. They had a prime photo op with a larger-than-life, pastel-colored chair in the middle of an Easter display. In the photo, I look so small sitting on the chair. Because I needed to decompress and handle the stress of Daddy's death, I had four double drinks. It took most of the next morning to recuperate. I promised myself I would never drink that many doubles again!

Charles and I were in our hotel room, and I laid out a tarot spread. I was really missing Erick, so I asked the cards how he was doing. *Is he happy?* Charles wanted to video the reading. Afterward, he said, "You have to see this." There were many orbs flying around me—more than I have ever seen in other videos. I couldn't believe it! Seeing the orbs made me feel vindicated. Spirit is around me, and I'm guided, directed, and protected. I acknowledged what I saw, and it changed my life. *I have been given spiritual gifts I shouldn't waste by using substances to escape reality. I choose to leave them alone.*

After classes ended, Charles and I returned home. *I am going to make positive changes in my life.* I got things in order before my Mommy Makeover. When my surgery date arrived, alone in the pre-op room, I sat in deep thought. Erick was in my heart. I talked to him telepathically, told him that I will always love him, but that I was moving forward with my life—getting this makeover for me, so I can feel better about myself. I'll be a new woman, on my own.

The surgery went well, but it would take time to recover. My friend and colleague, Summer, took care of me and attended to my every need. After she returned to work, Samantha and another close friend, Corinne, cared for me over the next week. Within two weeks, I was walking over two miles a day.

Before Memorial Day weekend, I received a "like" from a man on a dating website who piqued my interest. I am attracted to and intrigued by smart men. *Sapiosexual.* I have allowed myself to be open to dating men who can carry an intelligent conversation, make me laugh, have common decency, and who are ambitious and nice. Yes, looks attract me, but I am a realist and don't want to be judged on looks. So I glance at photos but want a detailed profile that shows me the essence of who that person is. Many women want all their boxes checked, but I don't have a list. I go with my intuition.

On his profile, Luke described himself as a professional and humorous, smart and conversational. When I saw his educational level and saw that he had the same degree as Erick, it almost stopped me from reaching out, but I sent a message. He replied and gave me his cell number. I chose to communicate through the site's messaging system for safety.

With a cell number, you can find information on the Internet. Having Luke's name and number allowed me to find him. He is a former man of the cloth but fell from grace by having a sexual relationship with a church member. He and Erick are of the same faith. *Are you freaking kidding me...they have the same educational degree and faith...synchronicity. Will I meet him?* My profile shows I'm "spiritual and not religious." *Did he read my information?* I didn't tell him I knew who he was, as I preferred to speak with him... *Will he be honest?*

It was Memorial Day. I looked forward to meeting him. We agreed to an upscale sports bar. *Really...another sports bar?* When I arrived, he was waiting outside, sitting on a dark metal bench. When he stood up, my first thought was, *You're shorter than your profile stated.* The inside of the bar was warm and welcoming; the walls and benches were rich, dark wood. Luke had beautiful, light blue eyes that reminded me of my grandpa's eyes. I felt his warmth and kindness. We walked inside and began the familiar dance of introduction and sharing details of our lives. It turns out that Luke not only had the same degree as Erick, but he'd gone to graduate school and obtained a master's degree. Our conversation flowed. His intelligence and humor drew me in.

I rarely tell my story first, but I wanted to give him a chance, and to see if my non-religious beliefs would scare him. I talked about spirituality and told him who I was. He didn't blink an eye when I said I read tarot cards. Luke told me our paths had been different, and he divulged the information I had found online. *How difficult his journey had been!* Neither of us judged the other's mistakes. He was expressive and intelligent, with a great sense of humor.

At the end of our date, Luke walked me to my vehicle and asked if he could kiss me on the cheek, and I let him. *No electricity.* Back at home, I cried. Luke had triggered me because I saw similarities between him and Erick. I drank a half-bottle of rum, just to sort it out in my mind. *I take two steps forward and one back with my Twin Flame path.*

Chapter 12
Healing Retreat

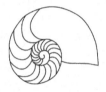

Luke and I got to know each other more. I loved that he could quote *Little House on the Prairie*. My comfort level with him came easily; we had a wonderful rapport. Our conversations were sweet and insightful. Luke is highly educated (I'm not), but he said he was enamored with me.

He came to see me and we had a long lunch. He kissed me. I can't explain what his kiss did to me—I couldn't quite put my finger on it. It was as though I had something in my throat. I went to the lake seeking clarity for the after-effects of his kiss. It was as if someone had sprinkled fairy dust on me, and I was looking through a thin spiritual veil. It sounds crazy, but it happened.

All was going well between us. After Luke and I had been seeing each other for a few weeks, he wanted to come over. I sensed how passionate he felt towards me, and he was not shy about telling me his intentions. He came over on a Friday at lunchtime, and we ended up in my bedroom. The sex was fun, happy, full of emotion—and intense! We had Divine transcendent sex. *Orgasm was powerful; different.* I'd never expected to have a relationship with a former preacher, much less have sex with one. *It was mind-altering and triggered something within me.*

Ten minutes after Luke left, I was standing in my bedroom and caught an image forming in the mirror. It was purples and blues that started in a nautilus shape and became larger. I rubbed my eyes… *Am I really seeing this?* The nautilus shell expanded—it looked like a DNA double-spiral helix. I watched, trying to absorb the image, and after a few minutes, it dissipated. *What did I just see?* I reached out to Luke. He had no explanation.

After researching online, I discovered I had seen a Fibonacci spiral, which is related to the Fibonacci sequence, and the Golden Ratio. I needed more information. I researched and discovered that the Golden Ratio is a mathematical ratio found in nature and art, the universe, and in many everyday designs that are pleasing aesthetically. There was a lot to ponder, but I had an upcoming trip to plan for.

Last fall, I was looking for a spiritual place to interact with other like-minded people. I did an Internet search for a Divine Feminine retreat and found the "Dragonfly Experience" offered by Felicia Grant, a spirit medium, reiki master, and soul coach. It was what my heart and soul needed.

I made plans to attend a small retreat held at Elohee (EL-oh-HEE) Center in Sautee Nacoochee, Georgia. Looking at the website, I saw they held the retreat within the Blue Ridge Mountains. Those mountains hold a special place in Erick's heart, and I wanted to see them. Melissa wanted to go with me.

Melissa and I had different spiritual wants and needs for the trip. On Thursday, after a very long drive, we arrived in the Blue Ridge Mountains range. We saw the beautiful Ocoee River against the vast cumulus clouds and felt the warmth of the bright sun. With my first glimpse of the majestic mountains, I was elated. We pulled over at the Hogpen Gap overlook. I stepped outside to take in the mountains, ridges, knobs, and gaps. I saw the varying shades of blue on the canvas before me. Joyful tears filled my eyes. *Erick had wanted us to travel here and stop at an overlook to make love.*

At one point in the trip, Melissa and I realized the GPS was no longer working. I was thankful I hadn't made this trip alone because I struggle to read a map. The road to Elohee is winding, and I envisioned Chris on a motorcycle snaking through the sharp curves—that image made my heart smile.

When we reached our destination, Eve Cook, who co-owns Elohee Center,[7] greeted us at the entrance. We parked at the bottom of a steep driveway in a makeshift parking lot. As a staff member shuttled us to the Eucalyptus cottage, we took in the serenity of the place. Our simple room was comfortable and provided everything we needed for our stay. We explored the complex, and I knew I would get my exercise on the uneven grounds. The Tea Room was open 24/7. Mandala Hall has seventeen sides, and its name means both "circle" and "center." It's the heart of Elohee and serves as the primary meeting space. Its windows overlook forest and valley. The cafeteria is at the lower level, where the center's nutritious food is served.

Melissa and I walked the grounds and admired the natural pond outside Mandala Hall. Stones and greenery surrounded the clear water pond, and I looked forward to drinking in the mountain views while dipping my toes in the pond. We would be in Mandala Hall for our introduction and Circle Time. Crystal Bowl Sound Healing would follow, with Tony, a sound therapy practitioner who is also a gifted medium. I looked forward to the session because the continual buzzing in my ears subsides only when I hear ocean waves, rushing water, or the vibration of a sound bowl.

---

[7] www.elohee.org.

We sat in yoga chairs on the polished wooden floor of Mandala Hall. Each person received a spiritual card, and mine was Believing in Magic, "True magic is abounding in my life!" At that moment, I felt it. Felicia Grant was our leader and introduced herself to our group of fifteen women. She has taken part in and led many retreats.[8] Our task was to greet another participant, ask about them, and share with the group.

After we completed circle time, Felicia encouraged us to relax while closing our eyes and listen to the art of sound healing. My ears quit buzzing as the melody began. The waves and pitch invigorated my soul. As we concluded our evening, a strawberry moon rose in the night sky. Her hue mesmerized me.

On Friday morning, we gathered in the tea room for our meditation session, which was to be followed by a guided nature walk. I sat in front of Felicia as the meditation began, thinking we were doing a relaxation meditation. As she began guiding us through a meditative release, I didn't realize this exercise would trigger my emotions about Erick. Non-stop tears ran down my hot cheeks. After the session ended, it was clear to me how attached I had been. *Oh my God, this agony is the feeling of letting go.* I knew I had to endure this unbearable pain. I realized that the grief of Erick's abandonment and rejection exacerbated my core wounds. As we concluded our session, I couldn't speak without crying.

We went on a guided nature walk, and although I was wearing sunglasses, I felt like the other women could read me—I felt naked. I was near the back of the line trying to collect myself—tears rolled down my face. Further into the walk, my tears slowed as we approached the statue of Ganesha, the elephant-headed Hindu god of success, beginnings, and prosperity. A few pieces of jewelry and trinkets adorned him.

We were on the red walking trail, identified by red hearts spray-painted on trees. The path narrowed at certain points,

---

[8] www.feliciagrant.com.

and we arrived at the meditation rocks. Melissa and I were alone and sat in silence, embracing the beauty and peace before us. As I meditated on the nature I saw and heard, I felt joy within my grieving heart.

Later that day, I walked into Mandala Hall and took in the room's essence. There were sound bowls of varying sizes and colors and many long glass windows. I lay on a mat in the center of the acoustically pleasing room. I still felt the pain from my meditation and felt tension in my body. A private sound-healing session would be followed by a massage. Tony, the practitioner, is a thin, soft-spoken man. He said that my heart, throat, and solar plexus chakras needed work, and that I was lacking playfulness in my life. When I allowed my barriers to drop, I absorbed energy from a tuning fork that Tony had placed on my ankle. I began seeing colors and shapes behind my closed eyes and felt jerks in my lower legs. The colors I saw in my third eye included vivid pinks and purples. I saw Egyptian hieroglyphs and an alien. At the end of my session, he said my chakras were clear, but that my throat chakra needed vocal work.

We had Circle Time with the group and Sound Healing. My spiritual card was Looking Deeper—"Deep within me is a majestic radiance." I knew it was true. We broke into groups of four. Each of us was to work on visualization and manifestation while sharing our energy. I felt connected to the strong women within my group. Each of us shared what we hoped to manifest for each person. As each person shared what they envisioned for themselves, we visualized our manifestation for them. I felt my Divine Feminine energy sitting in that circle. The women touched me, giving their abundance and love.

I was the last one to share what I desired. I told the group that I believe I am being Divinely guided to write about and share my Twin Flame journey. The book is meant to help heal activated Twin Flames who are new to the journey, but I hope it helps anyone who wants to heal. I explained that while I had thought union with my Twin Flame was the end game, now I realized part of the journey is about me healing my childhood traumas and core wounds. I felt empowered, uplifted, and unable to sleep.

Did the sound healing cause my awakened state? I walked outside in the moonlight to the Tea Room. The moon lacked some of the strawberry color from the previous evening, but it was still beautiful. I had brought my crystals to Elohee, and I let them charge under the moonlight.

It was peaceful on the mountain. I took my laptop to the Tea Room and wrote in healing solitude, asking God to allow the words to flow from my nimble fingers. I typed for two-and-a-half hours about Mama's death. When I tell people I lost Mama, I say that we both contracted COVID-19; she didn't make it, but I did. I know that I survived that adversity so that I could do my lightworker mission work and inspire others. With the biggest lump I've ever had in my throat, I said, "Mama, I miss you and love you." It hurt inside my heart.

Retreat members were free to wander the complex as we wished, and after I felt complete with my writing that morning, I left the Tea Room and joined Melissa in Mandala Hall. I felt drawn to a piece of photographic art that sat on the window seat. The image reflected what I'd seen in my bedroom mirror when Luke left my home—a nautilus shell, which grew in a spiral before my eyes. Melissa, aware of what I had seen at home, pointed to another photo. It depicted a row of bare trees with beautiful, earthy colors. In the center, there were two trees intertwined like a DNA strand. At the bottom, a Divine Feminine and Divine Masculine were naked and wrapped in each other's energy. I said to Melissa, "Holy crap." *More synchronicity.*

During another guided meditation, Felicia took us to an area in the forest where we visualized what we wanted to release. Spirit was guiding me to be strong so I could release Erick from my energy. *Let go of the pain and heal my broken heart.* I allowed myself to see Erick inside a clear bubble. I still wasn't ready to let him float upward, but I felt a big shift in the right direction.

After meditation, Melissa and I partnered with two women and together we went to see the 400-year-old Hemlock tree and the 100-foot waterfall along the walking trails. We grounded ourselves and transmuted negative energy by touching a tree. There were twenty small, inscribed stones at the bottom of the tree. I was speechless when I looked down and saw a stone with my twin's initials painted on it. Melissa pointed to a stone with Erick's name. She and I smiled at each other—another synchronicity.

Our small group proceeded to the waterfall near the Thanksgiving house. As we walked down the steep hobbit steps, I felt giddy with excitement. The waterfall has energetic healing properties, and its water rushes over varying levels of rocks and cascades 100 feet into a clear, peaceful, natural basin. We sat at the bottom of the waterfall and put our feet into the brisk water and sat. I felt my inner child coming out. Our group put our shoes on and climbed the hobbit steps and stone steps and went back to the grounds outside of Mandala Hall.

I sat outside on the stones surrounding the natural pond. After removing my shoes, I dipped my toes in the clear water amongst the plants and rocks and watched dragonflies land beside me in the pond. Looking at the horizon, I saw clouds framing the mountains. The clear blue sky gifted us with a perfect ending to our afternoon. I wanted to drink in every sight, smell, and touch I could before leaving.

In the evening, the ladies sat around the Fire Circle. Even though I take part in positive manifestation and release rituals each month, I don't know if others do this. While waiting for the ceremony to begin, I wrote eight things to manifest and seven to release. Felicia explained that each of us would feed the fire by throwing a bay leaf into the flame and read our intentions. She read hers first. I followed. One of my manifestations was to finish writing my manuscript by December 31. I threw my list at the fire, but it didn't reach the flame. I retrieved my list and threw it again, yelling, "Burn, bitch, burn." We all laughed.

Each woman verbalized her deepest wants and desires—this group of women will always hold a special place in my heart. After Felicia gave her final thoughts, I said, "I learned through my sound healing treatment that I need to be vocal. Can we scream around the circle?" She indulged me. We screamed. I finished by jumping up and down until no more sound came from my throat. The colors of the sky faded into late evening—they reminded me of the colors I'd seen during my sound healing session.

I was a different person than the one I'd been when I entered the retreat three days earlier. My internal vibration had increased. I felt happier than I had in years. I felt calm, knowing I had accomplished everything I'd intended for myself.

Melissa and I discussed how much personal growth we'd experienced. Everyone should make a trip to a retreat when their path becomes uncertain. As we prepared to sit for the last time, I saw my card: Acceptance. "I unconditionally accept, cherish, and love myself just as I am." *I do.* Our last circle time arrived. Felicia asked us to explain how things were different. Each of us gave a synopsis. When it was my turn, I said, "I haven't known peace in my life for a long time. This is the closest I have come." I looked at Felicia. "I am grateful," I said.

Circle time concluded by us moving closer together. Felicia makes a tradition of giving a stone to each attendee. We each received a beautiful, heart-shaped rose quartz crystal along with information about Archangel Chamuel, whose name means "He who sees God." His mission is to bring peace to the world, while protecting the world from fear, lower vibrations, and negative energies. We passed each crystal through the circle of hands and placed our manifestation and energy in each stone. I lost track of whose stone was whose, but each one carried my love, light, and positive energy. Our retreat over, Melissa and I packed and prepared to leave the peaceful mountain that had allowed me to ground myself and heal my heartbreak.

We stopped for a walk at Anna Ruby Falls, a dual waterfall in the Chattahoochee National Forest. Curtis Creek drops 153 feet and York Creek drops 50 feet to form twin waterfalls—*another synchronicity*. Because it's listed as an easy walk, I didn't put sneakers on, and made the mistake of walking in flip-flops. *OMG, what was I thinking! The Internet said it was just a half-mile.* My thighs burned as I neared the steep incline. Once we reached the top and saw the twin creeks merge and heard crashing water, I felt elated. The rushing water was a sight to behold. *So glad I did this.*

The trip had been more than I imagined it would be. It was food that nourished my soul. My spiritual growth was exponential. I radiated happiness. I realized I was on a natural high: *spiritual.* I hope to return to Elohee again when I need a boost to increase my internal vibration. Feeling peaceful, I smiled. I was moving forward with life.

Chapter 13

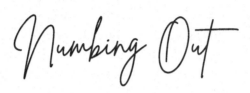

After my return from Elohee, Luke let me know how much he had missed me. "Are we okay?" he asked.

"Yes, we are!" My spiritual growth during the retreat had helped me. Luke was important to me. I had leveled up. We even made plans to fly to Las Vegas. He wanted to spoil me while we were there.

"I want to see you," Luke said.

Wanting to reconnect in multiple ways, I said, "I'm open."

"That sounds wonderful."

I was missing the retreat center. I felt connected to God there. I was excited—I had found myself again. My spiritual high continued. I lived in joy, my internal vibration high. Luke was happy I was in a better place. He texted to let me know how much he was thinking of me. I asked about his innermost thoughts. He wanted a slow, intimate, caressing, and passionate lovemaking session with me. *Yes!*

Early the next morning, I drove to see him. He opened the door to greet me with a sweet and passionate kiss and *looked* into my eyes. "I have missed you so much," he said. "I've fallen deeply in love with you."

He wanted to know how I felt. I let my barriers down and realized I loved him, too. I said those three words that change everything. Our passion erupted. When he said, "I love you," it felt pure. I told him I had only felt the same with one other person. Our lovemaking was intense. *Just the way I like it.* That morning was special—we both knew it. I loved the oneness and sensuality we shared. Luke agreed and said, "Sex with you was otherworldly." I felt deep intimacy with him; he is very sensual. Although his vibrational energy differed from Erick's, I could be in the moment with him. *Something I didn't expect.* I felt a Divine connection with him. I wondered if we might be a part of a spiritual monad.[9]

"What did you enjoy the most about the morning?" Luke asked.

I told him all of it, but that I especially enjoyed being in the moment. We planned to attend a family get together and spend the weekend together. He asked, "Does it mean I am a keeper if you are bringing me to meet family?"

"Yes," I replied.

A couple of days later, Luke began feeling sick. The next morning, he called and said he was feeling worse. After seeing a doctor, he called to say he had a sinus infection, and it had been treated with antibiotics and an injection. I knew an injection would produce excellent results in less time than antibiotic medication alone. My intuition alerted me, though: *Something is amiss.* "Do you feel better?" I asked. He said he was and was going to his sister's for a "low-key gathering."

I felt hurt. *Why isn't he going to come and be with me if he feels better?* My abandonment and rejection issues surfaced along with a fight-or-flight feeling: *instant anxiety.* I texted Luke. I saw myself repeating patterns and wouldn't be a part of them any longer. "This has triggered me and my core wounds," I told

---

[9] This is a term I have heard—it is more complex than I can explain—if you're interested in what it means, I recommend an Internet search.

him. "I had looked forward to seeing you and I understood the feeling under the weather. Before your illness, I thought the plan was for us to be together and I looked forward to getting to know you better. I thought when you started feeling better that we might at least see each other. An antibiotic shot helps you feel better in the first twenty-four hours. Family is important—and I know each person should be with them as time allows. But are you feeling differently about me? If yes, say so."

Luke responded, "I am not." *How could someone who confessed a deep love respond with just those three words?* I stewed on it, which caused a huge trigger to bubble to the surface. I needed to be around people. Considering our recent time together, I had told my friends about Luke. *Could I be wrong again? I thought we'd had a connection—but maybe he doesn't feel the same.* I tried not to dwell on it. But just below the surface, I felt afraid.

The morning after I texted Luke: silence. It triggered me in a way I hadn't experienced since Erick had ghosted me in the parking lot. I had irrational thoughts. I felt abandoned. I opened a bottle of vanilla rum and began to drink. I reached out to Samantha, and she warned me: "Don't text Luke." Alone, upset, and intoxicated, however, my drunken alter-ego reared its ugly head. In tears, I texted, "I am canceling my flight." Multiple drunken texts followed.

Luke replied, "I am dealing with a potential job change offer. I will call you later."

I sent more garbled texts. In the last one I asked, "It has nothing to do with me?"

All he replied was, "It's nothing. Please don't freak out."

Within an hour, I'd drunk almost an entire bottle of rum. I was inconsolable—once again in the pain body. Charles had called me earlier, and I reached out to him. He arrived. I was vomiting by this point. He stayed with me until I was less intoxicated. I fell asleep in my recliner in the late afternoon. I woke up four hours later, in the dark of night.

When I looked at my texts to Luke, shame set in. I texted him again and told him that he wasn't willing to talk to me or come over, and instead went to his sister's. This triggered my abandonment and rejection wounds. *He professed love, but again, I wasn't chosen.* The bitter truth in black and white was shocking. I felt empty. I said, "I don't do this, but when I extend my heart, it scares me. I am extending it as I haven't in so long." *How could I have been happy and then hit rock bottom within a few hours?!*

I walked over to my cabinet, retrieved the remaining rum, and poured it down the kitchen drain. Although I have experienced triggers, there were few of this intensity. In that instant, I promised myself I wouldn't ever do it again. The next morning, I awoke hungover. I licked my wounds. The previous day's events replayed in my mind. I was weepy.

The following day, I woke up mad as hell. It was time for my morning walk. I pray and walk with God daily and feel a divine presence around me. Mornings allow me to make strides towards becoming the best version of me, but I'm a work in progress. Instead of my normal peace, I felt angry at myself. I demanded answers from God. *Why does this keep happening to me? What do I keep doing wrong? Why can't I stop? Why am I triggered? I want to know.* Clairaudiently, I heard the words "numbing out." I realized I had repeated patterns and taken part in my *self-imposed* karma. Those two words hit home. I was repelled. I felt disgusted at myself.

After I returned home, I did an internet search to understand the inner workings of triggering. It's an emotional reaction which causes a psychological response to an upset in someone's life. Effects are found in war veterans, PTSD victims, depression, and other mental disorders. It was as though someone had slapped me in the face. I felt ashamed.

Numbing out is a harsh reality—and I'm a repeat offender. My emotions resulted because of deep emotional pain. I had tried to protect myself from the hurt that triggered me to become detached. Although I stay connected with the women in my life, I realized I had been using numbing out to keep romantic partners from getting close to my blocked heart chakra. Numbing was a protective barrier. I realized I had suffered from deep grief, depression, anxiety, and stress throughout the years. Two years ago, I weaned myself off depression medication, and I have felt more emotions than I have in twenty-five years.

I remembered Daddy's abuse of Mama. That trauma resulted in feelings that permeated me. When I feel abandoned, rejected, or triggered, I reach for alcohol to escape and to control the emotional, mental, and physical pain. I don't love the taste of alcohol, but I drink from the bottle—and numb out. All I want in those moments is to be held. I made a promise to God that I wouldn't numb out any longer. It didn't mean I wouldn't drink again, but I wouldn't teeter on the edge of a cliff any longer. I made peace with myself.

I messaged Luke. "I'm trying to do things differently," I said. "I'm sorry I texted you through my weakness. I couldn't understand what was going on from your side. We went from us communicating to it changing overnight. I don't understand why. I ask you through compassion to explain what went wrong—a week ago, you told me how much you missed and loved me. I wanted to know why it had changed so I could have closure."

Luke called. He said he was giving me time to calm down. "Are you an alcoholic?"

Me? An alcoholic? My guard went up. "No," I said.

Luke's first girlfriend was an alcoholic, and my actions had triggered him. We discussed it, and I told him I didn't do it intentionally. He said he was on his way to his interview and that we'd talk again. But then he ghosted me, just as Erick had done eighteen months before in the parking lot. That fight-or-flight feeling kicked in again.

The next few days weren't easy, but I was thankful to have an answer. I accepted the outcome more easily than I'd expected. Erick had come into my thoughts, and I realized his childhood wounds carried over into his adult life, too. I believe his traumas contributed to him becoming an alcoholic. I felt connected to him and realized: *Twin Flames mirror each other, and we do.* Looking into the night sky, I asked God to allow Erick to hear my words. Disgusted, I said, "You and I are both toxic. We need help."

The next evening, I sat in my chair and allowed my mind to relax. I was dozing off and received words clairaudiently: "Honey bee." I knew Erick had heard my words. Our telepathic link remained. We both needed to heal. Although I had just returned from Elohee two weeks earlier, I booked myself into another event at that peaceful mountain retreat for more healing and to write the heavier parts of my journey.

Since Elohee had brought me healing, I searched online again to find another Divine Feminine retreat. I found a Sacred Feminine Ayahuasca retreat in Orlando, Florida, that was scheduled for September. Ayahuasca was a word I hadn't heard until Erick mentioned he wanted to take part in a sacred ceremony with his son. I researched. It is a South American plant-based tea, also known as DMT, which produces a psychedelic response. I know the energetic cord between Erick and me is still active—and probably always will be, because that is the nature of a soul-based Twin Flame relationship—but

I hoped that Ayahuasca might help me release attachment to outcome in my Twin Flame journey.

On my way to Elohee's Rest and Relaxation weekend, I stopped in the Bavarian alpine town of Helen, Georgia. Helen is a small, charming tourist town. I went inner tubing for the first time in the Chattahoochee River, which flows through the middle of town. My shoe came off, and I got out of the inner tube and slipped on the slick rocks in the water. I strained the fleshy part of my right palm. *Ouch!* The water was cold in late July. After a couple hours, my floating trip ended, and I got in my car and drove to the hotel.

After checking into the hotel, I went to dinner and walked through town. At dusk, I returned to the hotel. GPS should have worked, as I had a strong cell tower connection, but it didn't, and I got lost on the streets in the dark. After an hour of walking, I made it back to the hotel.

In my hotel, I grabbed my car fob and room card to get my suitcase. When I returned to the room, my room card wasn't with me. I went to the front desk to get a new one. A couple arrived, and I let them go ahead of me. As I listened to their conversation, customer service made a statement about the new tattoo on the lady in front of me, which was covered in a clear dressing.

I looked at it, eyes wide. It was the Sacred Geometrical Fibonacci Spiral (nautilus spiral) I'd seen six weeks before in my home mirror. It was surreal. When I returned to my room, the room card was lying on the desk. My intuition alerted me: *the Divine had delayed me in returning to the hotel at the right moment so I could see that tattoo.* Everything happens in the right time, at the right place, for the right reason. I smiled and knew I needed to trust in the universe and let things flow.

Chapter 14

Releasing Attachment to Outcome

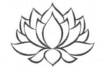

Mornings are when I connect with God. Not only do I pray, but I sense His loving presence and ask for guidance. My daily mantra is "Let me live in your light through your Grace, and help me do my highest good." Luke had returned recently to me. My trip to Soul Quest in Orlando to take part in the Ayahuasca ceremony was near, and I asked for continued guidance, direction, and protection. This was my third trip traveling alone—I was outside my comfort zone.

Although Ayahuasca is illegal in the United States, a religious waiver allows adult participants to engage in Ayahuasca ceremonies. It's also called Aya, and people use it to experience visions. It activates parts of the brain associated with memory, emotion, intention, and visual perception. People say it's like having multiple therapy sessions at once. There is a mystery surrounding Ayahuasca—I learned it doesn't always give what it's asked for, but it gives what's needed.

This was a Sacred Feminine Ayahuasca Ceremony, and most of the women there were first-time participants. We spoke about what the evening might bring. I walked into the narrow doors of the peaceful Maloka. Spiritual tapestries hung from the walls. There was a circular, lowered altar in the center of the room. There were volunteers, dressed in white clothing, and spiritual leaders who lifted us with inspirational words and prepared us for the ceremony through prayer and wisdom. I felt unity through sisterhood. What was given through Ayahuasca would become part of my soul.

Each of us sat cross-legged on a rectangular light mat. We were on a spiritual path and were encouraged to vocalize our intent for drinking Ayahuasca. As part of the ritual, we passed a wooden wheel that would be placed in the fire later and shared what we hoped to get from drinking Aya. As we each said what we desired, we wrapped our intentions with a thin yarn around the wheel. "First," I said, "I want to release attachment to the outcome with my Twin Flame, as closure has eluded and burdened me. Making a connection with my maternal ancestors is second. Last," I said, "I'm connected to Source and Divine, but I haven't heard my Spirit Guides and want to." When the last person's intention had been shared, a female shaman offered us rapè, a snuff.

Rapè can help relax a person who will drink Aya. My nerves were on edge and let me know I was far outside my comfort zone. I accepted the snuff to help me relax. A facilitator sat in front of me with a long tube and blew it into my nose. I had an immediate light-headed feeling, different from smoking marijuana. They provided a bucket for expelling the rapè from the mouth, because it's not to be swallowed. After thirty minutes of a relaxed state, we awaited our destiny with Aya.

Elders and volunteers spoke ceremonial words and let us know they would give us a small dose, just a tablespoon. At the end of two-hours, a gong would sound to mark the beginning of the journey. If anyone wanted an additional booster, it could be requested and received. The drink was a dark, plant-based liquid. I didn't want to smell it. *When I was younger, I would never have ingested a substance like this.* The practitioner touched my heart, blew upon me spiritually, and gave me a tablespoon of the Ayahuasca brew. I stepped forward for smudge cleansing.

I walked into a dark room. Above each tapestry on the wall was a strand of lights. They had encouraged us to bring family heirlooms. I wore jewelry that had belonged to Mama, Granny, and a great-grandmother. Next to my mat, I laid my Grandpa's shoehorn, my grandmother's Bible, my great-grandmother's snuff can, my Divine Feminine and Divine Masculine orgonites, a Phenacite crystal, and two Shiva Lingam stones. Against my chest I laid Erick's business card, a piece of paper from our casino trip, and a honey bee orgonite.

The shaman gave us approval to ingest our Ayahuasca medicine. Squeezing my nose, I chugged a tablespoon of bitter, horrendous substance. *Indescribable.* I swished water in my mouth twice and spit it out before the smell and taste came together. I propped myself against the wall, put my eye mask on, and waited for Aya to show me her effects. *I prayed. Let me live in Your love and light.*

A woman swaddling her newborn eased us into the journey by singing spiritual songs. The one out-of-place song was "You Are So Beautiful to Me." I caught myself holding my breath—this was a song Erick had texted to me. I felt it had been sent from his higher self.

After two hours, I heard a gong. Through closed eyes, I saw the face of a Native man. My journey began. I found myself inserted into the Universe. Images, patterns, numbers, and energy rushed towards me in oranges and yellows, as if they were part of a roller coaster. I saw religious symbols. A cross made of pure light appeared, and I realized that Luke had experienced multiple religious incarnations. The name "Jacob" came to me, and I felt that Luke was connected to the biblical Jacob.

I also knew that I'm meant to feel deep love in my life by giving and receiving. The space I experienced was expansive. My mind couldn't comprehend what I saw. I was a small fragment within the stars; a minute particle of energy within the Universe. In a kaleidoscope of colors and images, I felt invigorated. I was at home and didn't want to leave the imagery I saw.

Four people came into my energetic field: Charles and I were connected through other lifetimes, Chris was a protector, and Melissa was a comfort during my journey. One person made no sense—I saw the face of a woman I identified as Lily Potter, Harry Potter's mother. Towards the end, I yawned and told God my physical body was tired. I was one with the Universe.

As I came down from my journey, still feeling the effects of Aya, I waddled outside the lodge, looked into the sky, and saw many stars. I joined others around the fire pit to share my experience. I was happy and felt on fire with knowledge. Each participant shared their journey, and I realized that my experience had differed from the others'. They shared their heartaches and activated my empathy. I wished I could take the pain from them. Although far from healed, I had done self-care and healing work for over two years. If I hadn't, my Ayahuasca journey wouldn't have been such a wonderful experience.

Looking into the sky, I saw a bright star with three smaller ones clustered around it. I felt connected to the Universe and knew beyond a doubt that I had originated from a star system and have incarnated multiple lifetimes. It felt familiar. *Remembrance.*

It was late—after 3:00 a.m.—when we went to our rooms. I was on a spiritual and emotional high. I wanted to speak to Luke, but it was too late. A few journeyers continued into the night—they wouldn't take part in the daytime ceremony. Their bodies couldn't take another round of Ayahuasca.

The following morning, I rested and enjoyed the silence in the Maloka before joining the others outside. I caught the end of restorative yoga under shade trees with hints of sunshine peeking through the branches. We were at ease. We lay on multi-colored rugs, a white bucket next to each of us. It was in the mid-80s when the afternoon ceremony began, and I was not looking forward to chugging the medicine in hot weather.

The items I had with me on this day were my grandmother's Bible, memorabilia of Erick, and metaphysical stones. I wore the eye mask from the night before and closed my eyes. I allowed my journey to begin. The melodic songstress lulled me into my daytime experience. I heard a lady with acute anxiety screaming, "Make it stop! Make it stop! Make it stop!" She was having a rough journey. Knowing that Aya's effects can't stop after you drink, my heart went out to her. Some women vomited and purged. I hoped I wouldn't.

I allowed my journey to come organically. We received the same notification that we could take a booster if we wanted. I asked for an additional one-half tablespoon. Somehow I tasted it more, and I winced. *Gross. I didn't think it could taste worse than last time.* I lay down, expecting a full-on psychedelic experience, but found myself in a peaceful space. I removed my mask and was aware of my surroundings in 3D, yet I felt I was part of another dimension. There is a thin veil between time and space and between the physical and spirit worlds. I believed I was in the Garden of Eden. I was under an enormous tree—the Tree of Knowledge. I asked God for answers about my Twin Flame journey and waited for Erick's higher self. Tears flowed from my eyes and what my mask did not absorb flowed down my face. The volunteers placed an umbrella over me to shield my fair skin from the bright sunshine. I asked, "Who am I?" and the name "Lilith" dropped into my thoughts. Lilith was Adam's first wife, and I believe I am a modern-day incarnation of Lilith. *She is misunderstood.* I saw a dark shadow of a man, but it didn't scare me. I knew he was Adam. The blackness transformed into a bright white light that represented Luke. I was upside down on a cross and felt no pain. Clairaudiently, I heard, "It's all washed away." I was emotional.

I felt sweat pouring from my face mixing with my tears. *My purging.* Erick's energy crept into mine and Luke's. *Is Erick trying to tell me that Luke is my Twin Flame?* My weeping continued. It was a spiritual experience. I felt Erick's love and saw Harry Potter's mother, Lily. *Why is she here? It makes no sense!* I heard Lily say, "Sweetheart, you're ready. Let go." I tried to understand what was happening and causing me pain. My intuition told me it was Erick's higher self telling me, "Let go of attachment to outcome with me and our Twin Flame journey." I purged more tears. It took every bit of love I felt to do the unimaginable. A tall white wall melted away, and I felt Erick's full love handing me to Luke. I accepted this. The word SHARE came through, and I knew I would finish my book. I couldn't hide anymore. I was to share my journey. It cemented the book title of my labor of love—I'd had the courage to release and allow myself to love again with an open heart.

I could do what had once been unimaginable. I placed Erick inside a clear bubble and let go. It was the hardest thing I've ever done. I released him fully. I heard clairaudiently, "I am love." I felt inner peace for the first time in my life. Looking at the tree branches I could see beyond the umbrella, I saw the Flower of Life, a sacred geometry pattern, and realized I was coming down from my journey. The total journey lasted six hours.

As I left the ceremonial space, I placed Erick's business card in my bucket. There's so much I'd tried to understand. I accepted what I'd experienced. There was a closing ceremony, but I'd journeyed much longer than others, and didn't attend. Instead, I sat on the patio and allowed the events to replay in my mind. Volunteers were available if needed. At group integration in the Lotus Lodge, a counselor offered support as we shared our journeys. It was an exhausting yet fulfilling day.

After integration, I experienced a vision. Luke was in my home, bathing me and caring for me. He washed my hair. *Did I just see that?*

It was time to go home. I asked Luke to pick me up from the airport and felt him tremble when he hugged me. He is a gentle, loving man, and I knew that is why Erick showed me I could release the Twin Flame journey in earnest and open my heart to new love.

I told Luke what happened on Friday night but couldn't tell him about the daytime ceremony until he'd read a rough draft of the section of my book that described my combustible, soul-connection affair with Erick. Luke had to understand what it meant for me to tell him my heart was open after Erick (which I never thought could happen). For Luke to accept me, I had to be honest. I had to share my imperfections, mistakes, and the chain of events that are part of me.

The Ayahuasca experience exhausted me. I wanted to shower and turned on the water for it to heat. I stepped inside and closed my eyes. Luke surprised me when I opened them. I screamed. *I'm still jumpy. Aya is still in my system. We were told its effects would continue after our return home.* Luke bathed me gently and washed my hair. *Clairvoyance.* He left to go home. It felt good to sleep in my bed at home.

At 3:00 a.m., I woke up. I remembered a dream. I was thirty feet above the ground and stood upon a stairway, levitating in the air, while looking down. Erick and two other people were at the bottom of a set of steps. He looked up at me. There was a white wall to the left of the steps, and the people pulled Erick around the corner where he couldn't see me.

Less than twelve hours later, I took a nap and remembered a second dream. I was in a dark room at the local country club, dressed casually. There were many tables with well-dressed people sitting around them. I had to walk through the room. Although I couldn't see Erick or Karen, I sensed them in the blackened room. I heard her voice say, "V.C. Pitt."

Although I have vivid lucid dreams, these were different. When I awoke, I felt no attachment to the outcome with my twin. Aya gave me not only what I'd wanted but what I'd needed. *How could this happen?* I'm not sure. I felt light for the first time in over three years and still felt Ayahuasca in my system. I was floating and emotional when I shared my spiritual experience with those closest to me.

Not long after my return, Luke ghosted me for a second time. *Was it me telling him that his father was the CEO at the business where Erick's grandmother and my Aunt Lauren worked? Did he recognize how unlikely it would be for Erick, he, and I to have a link through family members at one place of employment, at the same time over thirty years ago? Was it what he'd read about the affair?* This ending didn't trigger me as it had in July. I reached out to Chris and asked, "What do I keep doing wrong?"

He said, "You need to listen to me. He isn't strong enough for you." *Could Chris be right?*

Despite difficulties in my romantic life, I choose myself. Two years ago, a professor told me I am self-actualized at the top of Maslow's Hierarchy of Needs, but until now, I didn't agree. Whatever spiritual opportunity presents itself to me in the future, I am open to it. I invite all possibilities and embrace who I am.

Chapter 15
Evolving Divine Feminine

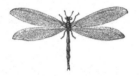

I was unprepared for how my life would change over four years. I often reflect on my life since my spiritual awakening and embrace the changes through the light and darkness of my Twin Flame journey. In my youth, I was a sweet person. But in adulthood, I became an unhappy, hardened, Type-A person. I made some poor choices, and my childhood and adult wounds and traumas surfaced. I have reconnected with the good parts of who I am and have come full circle—I'm like I was in my early twenties, but a better version. I'm more at peace.

As I mentioned earlier, a few years ago, I began listening to tarot readings on YouTube and had a few sessions with tarot readers and intuitive mediums. People connected with religion think of tarot in a negative light, but I view it as a divination tool. I was drawn to the cards in my early twenties, but because they intimidated me, I didn't keep the set I purchased. After I divorced, I bought the Rider-Waite deck and a book explaining the different energies of the cards. In less than three years, my tarot and oracle collection has grown. Some decks I connect with and receive clear messages from; others I don't keep. As a reader, I tap strongly into love energy. My intuition has increased, and readings I do for others reveal hidden secrets.

Two years ago, I received a Past Life Regression. I remembered three lifetimes that had occurred in the last 400 years. One of those memories involved being in a white wooden house over 100 years ago. I was a young teen, dancing with a boy in overalls to music from a Victrola. In my second life, I was a Native American and attached to Erick as a tribal chief. In the last one, Erick was married to me and had an affair with Karen that ended with me taking my own life. It was painful to remember that I had ingested a poisonous substance, and to see myself lying on a bed with Erick holding me as I slipped away. I felt as if an elephant was sitting on my chest. *Will Erick and I ever get it right in 3D?*

Later that year, I had an Akashic Records reading. The Akashic Records is a library in the non-physical plane of archives and memories (events and knowledge) of each soul's thoughts, purpose, ideas, and actions that are part of our past, present, and future. My record includes that I'm from Mintaka, part of Orion's belt. It is the star system I came from, my primary and secondary Archangelic realm of training (which includes compassion, nurturing, tolerance, growth, and success for this life), and it provided my soul's primary purpose (being present). My record included my current and strongest intuitive gift (clairsentience) and my empathic gifts (medical and emotional, and my experience with crystals) and the wounds I carried into this lifetime. I have lived through several periods of history, which explains why I am drawn to Eastern beliefs instead of traditional religion. The information I received reflects experiences and lessons in this lifetime.

A year later, I had a second Akashic reading that showed I am making progress in this lifetime. I will have another update in the future.

When I became conscious of being a Twin Flame, I first thought it was just a romantic connection with spiritual aspects—but I was wrong. Many people think they are their lover's twin, but they romanticize the idea—their experiences could be soulmate or karmic lessons, or part of a soul contract. Being a Twin Flame challenges you—the relationship is for individual soul growth. In my Twin Flame soul contract lessons, I included abandonment, rejection, and issues of self-worth.

Signs and synchronicities continue to come to me daily, through meditation, dreams, music, and Angel numbers. Erick's life path number is 7, and mine is 9. Seventy-nine is a number I've seen since I began working in healthcare administratively on 8/8/88. Our Angel team and spirit guides give us numbers as signs and symbols that, when deciphered, give us direction for our lives. An Internet search gives descriptions,[10] and it's up to each person to interpret signs and synchronicities for their highest good.

Erick awakened me, and his actions affected me because we mirror each other. Think of it as being on a seesaw, trying to find a balance between masculine and feminine energies. Once I realized our deep connection, I knew that if both of us were in a lower vibration, neither of us had a chance. If I didn't start healing and changing our path, we would remain unhealed and in the pain body. One twin works harder than the other at healing—usually it's the twin who identifies as the Divine Feminine who steps up to the plate.

I called things off five times when Erick and I were involved, but he wouldn't let me go until the affair came out. He chose tradition, ego, and pride. I believe he stays married because of his fear of financial loss through divorce and what family, friends, and his clients will think. He once told me he would be a poor

---

[10] https://www.ask-angels.com/spiritual-guidance/angels-and-numbers/#chapter7. https://www.angelmessenger.net/the-ultimate-guide-to-angel-numbers-and-their-meanings/. https://www.ryanhart.org/angel-numbers/.

bastard if he divorced. I have tried to reconcile how a couple stays together without genuine love being part of the equation.

When our affair was discovered, Erick was a coward. I didn't want to acknowledge it, but now I can: I know I reflect him through my past fears. Although I love him, it's with healthy boundaries. He remains married, but I have felt his energy and have connected with him through dreams. This year, I moved forward, to focus on my healing and to accept that the link to our twin is never completely severed in this lifetime—because we are two parts of the same soul. Emotional triggers lessen as time passes. It took over three years to release expectations of outcome in my Twin Flame journey.

My magnetic connection with Erick brought me to my knees and sucked me into darkness, but I persevered. I know I am guided, directed, and protected by the Divine, Spirit, and the Universe. I wish I could say my journey has a storybook ending, but real life isn't a fairytale.

There were truths about myself I faced throughout my journey. I was codependent, but my self-worth is no longer linked to my job or material success, or what others think or say about me. Rejection is painful and is something I still try to avoid. Abandonment has brought me to my knees many times over.

Good and bad karma are real. I am trying to resolve what I can so it doesn't follow me into my next lifetime. I don't want to carry negativity into my next incarnation. I want blessings, not karmic lessons. Most recently, I resolved karma that required me to swallow my ego and my pride. I take part in new moon manifestation and full moon release, and I manifest positivity and release burdens. During both cycles for many months, I manifested that karma is resolved between Erick, Karen, Greg, and me. I have prayed to God that he grant me forgiveness for my actions that caused Greg and Karen pain, as I did many things wrong in my past. Kurt, Roman, and Ryan's lives were impacted by the affair. I can never apologize enough to them, but I am deeply sorry for how it affected their lives. *I have so much regret.*

Several people have said to me, "You are a good person despite having been through a lot." It's by persevering through adversity that we face hurt and heartache, learn our lessons, and overcome our challenges. In the past, I viewed myself as weak and didn't think I could be strong. It's a choice you have to make when there is no other way. I have mostly healed myself and have become very strong. Others notice my transformation.

I wasn't vulnerable in the past, but now I am open to others seeing the real me; who I am. I have found my inner Divine Feminine strength and no longer live from a wounded worldview.

Self-care and healing assist us in loving ourselves. How can others love us if we don't love ourselves? When I began my journey in November four years ago, I saw my physical and internal flaws. Erick allowed me to see myself through his eyes. Today, I look at myself as an average woman in my fifties who is becoming the best version of herself, and I hope to inspire others through unconditional love. A continual work in progress and twice divorced, I'm receptive to a high-level soulmate coming into my life when a higher power brings them in, in Divine timing.

Two years ago, at the beach I saw a Merkabah. I saw a sacred geometry shape for the third time last summer. The primal energetic force I felt deepened my thirst for spiritual learning, and I hope to continue to learn and to share my knowledge and experience with others.

This year allowed me to find retreats in alignment with my spiritual path, including Elohee and Ayahuasca. I will take part in three retreats next year, including a return trip to Soul Quest to drink Aya. This time, it's about me and what remains to be discovered. I will return to Elohee in April. There are plans for a September retreat in Sedona, one of the biggest metaphysical hubs in the United States. I have also researched and taken part in alternative healing. I've received reiki clearings. (Reiki is an energetic healing technique that originated in Japan and keeps Chi energy flowing)

When I returned to Elohee in October, my sound healing session confirmed my progress over four months. On the last night at Elohee, our leader, Felicia, led a sacred fire circle and played her Native American drum. She performed a reiki session on me. It was peaceful, and she played a dolphin meditation near my right ear. As I relaxed and she began clearing my chakras, I felt coolness on my left ear—it was reminiscent of the night Mama almost died. The dolphin meditation changed by itself to Native American chanting and drum beating. It was unexplained. I asked if someone was near my left ear, and Felicia saw a Native American man and received a channeled message: *I am a beacon of light to others.* The lights flickered from supernatural energy in that room.

My morning walks allow me to connect with God daily. Through prayer, I do my highest good identifying as an empathic lightworker who is a Twin Flame Divine Feminine. I ground myself at an older oak tree and leave negativity, anxiety, fear, sadness, doubt, worry, and illusion at the tree, and allow it to transmute the energy into love and light. My spiritual path hasn't been easy, but inner strength allows me to trust in the fluid process. I try to understand situations that happen to me through God's love and light.

My spiritual gifts include clairsentience, clairaudience, claircognizance, and clairvoyance. I first felt clairsentience, my gut feeling, when I was in my teens. It has served me well. My clairaudience began three years ago. I receive the Divine and Erick's messages through lyrics from 1970's songs. I have experienced claircognizance and clairvoyance a few times. Channeling is newer for me. I hope my gifts continue to grow.

I have made mistakes and repeated patterns. But now, I make different decisions, resulting in better outcomes. It turns out I was my worst enemy for many years. Now I handle situations through love. I live in my truth. Unconditional love is my greatest gift. It's something I have experienced with the birth of my children and three romantic partners, all of whom have helped me know I'm lovable—and that has allowed me to love myself.

I hope that through my story I can inspire others starting their Twin Flame journeys so they don't feel alone or hopeless. There were many times I wanted to give up, but friends and family loved and supported me during my darkest hours. God carried me when I wasn't able to walk. Now, I trust and have faith that the Divine will bring what's in my highest good.

Where do I go from here? My future is unwritten, but I see myself guided towards a healing shaman path, which will help others. Over time, the transition will happen. I have learned patience. My childhood and adult wounds and my traumas no longer define me. The Divine has brought people into my life only to remove them, but I trust the process and live in peace. I am a survivor and look forward to what my future holds as I develop.

I hope my story inspires you to begin your own healing path. I hope it is viewed as a reference to help anyone, Twin Flame or not, to heal through adversity, loss, and pain. There is light at the end of the dark tunnel.

Epilogue

Brian left me a voice message I found months after it was left. I'm not sure if he was on drugs. He spewed anger. He said he didn't care if I liked the message or not, that I was a piece of shit because I'd messed him over with Mama (regarding his exclusion from her estate) and because I didn't go to Daddy's funeral. Even though he hated Daddy, he went. He told me he hates me and hopes I die a miserable death. I choked back tears and disbelief.

I no longer consider Brian my brother. I pity him but will not open myself up to his anger or allow toxic people into my life. Other extended family members continue to support and love me.

I was recovering from Brian's angry tirade and working on my book revisions. The Divine pushed me to finish the book before the end of December. I was relieved to have finished my labor of love with time to spare.

Earlier in the month, I had a mammogram, which resulted in an ultrasound. The doctor wanted to do a biopsy of my left breast. No biggie; I've had to go back different times because I have fibrocystic breasts and sometimes images are not clear. I'd had a breast biopsy before, where the doctor didn't see a need to remove a lump. Lying on the cold table waiting for the biopsy, I looked at the on-screen image. It was taller than it was wide, a solid black area that looked similar to radiological photographs of the colon. When I asked the location of the spot, I was told it was in the three o'clock position. *Gulp, that's a different spot than the one before.* The radiologist placed titanium clips inside my breast, in case any doctors needed to find it in the future.

It was the holiday season, so it was close to a week before I received my results. Working in the field of healthcare as I do, I've learned the inner workings of when to worry. No news is good news. The following day, a doctor I work with asked me to come in to discuss my biopsy results. *I have breast cancer.* That afternoon, Melissa and I saw my doctor, who confirmed my intuitive thought. Nothing prepares you to be told you have invasive ductal carcinoma. *Oh shit.* A lot of things go through your mind when you are told you have malignant cancer—everything from *Oh my God, I'm going to die,* to *I might have to go through surgery or have chemo and/or take radiation,* to *what it will cost?* There are many more thoughts, but you get the idea.

Over the next three days, I went through all stages of grief except denial and anger. Many people wouldn't agree with me, but I realized that my sickness is something I chose as part of my soul contract before my incarnation to Earth. Kurt didn't respond when I texted him. It was hard telling Roman, but he was supportive. I am grateful.

On the third day after receiving the news, New Year's Day, I was weepy and sad. I looked upward and told God, "I'm scared." I didn't want to die alone. *Is this it for me? If yes, I accept my fate. If not, please let me live. Please let me only have a lumpectomy. Let it be contained to the breast with no lymph involvement, and no chemo or radiation.* I faced my mortality.

Three things happened within an hour that afternoon. I pulled three Sacred Oracle cards, which included that I should surrender to the power of prayer (*miracles can happen*), release my burdens, and use my intuition by looking beyond the surface (i.e., listen to my inner voice). A physician I work with texted me words of inspiration and told me, "You'll beat this!" He had faith. A lady from my first Elohee retreat sent me a text with a photo telling me that a candle had been lit for me in the National Lutheran Church in Reykjavik, Iceland. As a former breast cancer survivor, she hoped I'd stay in the light. I broke down and cried, accepted my situation, and told God, "No matter what, I trust and have faith."

One week after my diagnosis was confirmed, I had my appointment with a breast surgeon. During an ultrasound, she saw my lymph area was congested. *Has it spread to my lymph nodes?* Bloodwork, an MRI, and gene testing were the following week. She gave me the choice of a mastectomy or lumpectomy with radiation. *Thank God I have a choice.* I had surgery in mid-January, three weeks after my diagnosis, to remove the cancer and the surrounding lymph nodes.

My surgery was a walk in the park compared to my Mommy Makeover surgery. The final measurement of my tumor was 2.1 cm high by 1.9 cm wide. Almost an inch high, it was aggressive (score 8/9) and poorly differentiated, but was contained to just the breast. *OMG, did I hear her right?* I would have a catheter device inserted for ten rounds (twice daily for five days) of partial irradiation, which was targeted internal radiation. My heart and lungs were more protected by using this method.

When I saw the catheter device, reality set in. It was bigger than I thought it would be, and the part to be inserted in my breast looked like a beater on a hand mixer. Panic set in. Lots of tears. To be honest, I struggled more with the idea of the insertion than surgery. *You will put your big girl panties on for this.*

The day before radiation started, I was due to have the device inserted. A medical assistant gave me a valium. I had elevated anxiety and tried to relax. My blood pressure was through the roof. I was terrified. I cried, knowing I would be awake as my breast was sliced open and the catheter was fitted inside me.

I sat alone in the exam room waiting for the valium to take effect. I had asked others through social media to pray for me at the time of the appointment, and I prayed to God, too. Before the doctor came in and gave me several injections of lidocaine, I went into a meditative state. As I sat there, faces of people I had asked to pray for me—friends, classmates, family—appeared in front of me, being shuffled towards me like a deck of cards. It brought me peace.

I thought about Erick. I knew that if I'd called out to him through the ethers, his Divine Masculine would rescue me. But I knew too that I was okay on my own—*I can do this*. Still, I was terrified, and couldn't stop my tears. *I feel like a caged animal.* The procedure was over quickly and, since I was numbed, I only felt a tugging sensation. But it's one of the hardest things I've ever had to do.

Friends and family drove me to each radiation treatment. The spots and flecks that I see and know are Angels were in the room with me as I received ten treatments. *I was not alone.* My doctor says I'm cancer free, but I prefer the term "no evidence of disease." Tiredness kicked in two weeks after the radiation ended. I remained tired for about a month, but I'm grateful and doing well! Soon I will take an estrogen-blocking medication since my cancer was hormone driven.

My total time from mammogram to the catheter removal was seventy-seven days. Most people who see me can't believe I had cancer—I don't look sick. I have survivor's guilt because so many other people have harder treatment plans, where surgery may not be an option. They have longer radiation, or months of sickening chemotherapy, and some don't make it. I am grateful to have been blessed with very little treatment. My heart is full.

I can't end this book before I give you an update on other things that have happened. In March, two weeks after the radiation ended, Luke came back into my life. I had reached out to him for prayer during my cancer ordeal. The last chapter of my book made him cry. He couldn't figure out why he was emotional about it, and I explained he felt the unconditional love I have for him. Luke felt that God had hugely impactful plans for me after reading it. He told me he still loved me and wanted to marry me. Luke wanted to take care of me. If we weren't to marry, he wanted me as a friend in his life.

I was guarded, and rightfully so. After a month, Luke ghosted me again. This time it was different, as I knew I had done nothing to warrant his unacceptable behavior. I called him out on it, told him he had lied, that what he'd done was shitty, and that I didn't deserve it. "What would you do if someone treated your sister like you treated me?" I asked.

He acknowledged my anger and disappointment. He said it was justified, and he wanted to speak with me. Luke said, "I don't let people in when I am experiencing difficulties." This time I didn't answer him. I ghosted him. I did the right thing for myself. I don't regret it.

As I moved forward with my life, I returned to Soul Quest for two additional Ayahuasca ceremonies. Both nights revealed my strong Divine Feminine energy close to God/Source. During both journeys, I felt my soul's forever connection to my Twin Flame. After the first ceremony, for the first time in months, my throat chakra activated. It was a confirmation that we connected during the ceremony. I was given a message that my future includes hands-on healing using crystals, which confirmed my earlier Akashic Record Reading as a Crystal Empath. I saw purples and green on a ribbon with dots inside. Those dots represent light codes within me that are waiting to be activated. The second time, like the first, I was given a message "You are love," but this time, "You are pure and special" also came through. It was a fulfilling experience. I will go back in the distant future for more soul-purpose information through more Ayahuasca journeys.

As I mentioned earlier, before my divorce was final, I saw a psychic medium. I went back to the same psychic recently for an updated reading. As I entered her office, she'd already written down an outline of what she'd received from her Spirit Guides about me: I would do hands-on healing (which reinforced what Ayahuasca had shown me: that I would help heal others), and that my book will be released in a few months, but that it will take time for it to reach the people it is supposed to help. *I am patient.*

The number of channeled songs I receive has increased. My connection with Erick and his higher self through dreams remains strong. Meditation brings images of he and I in past lives. Signs and synchronicities happen often, so I don't dwell on them. I go with the flow. Crystals and stones are now part of who I am, which has helped my psychic development. Oh, and work got better! The horrible manager I dealt with was let go by the physician of the large practice to which I provide contracted services. God takes care of things in his timing.

Melissa and I returned to Elohee in April to attend another Felicia Grant Dragonfly Retreat. Elohee is beautiful in the spring. The flowers were in full bloom, and we reconnected with a few friends from the first retreat. My editor returned an edited draft of my manuscript, and I completed many of the revisions at Elohee. As I left the Blue Ridge Mountains, I knew how blessed I was to be living and enjoying life.

In June, I will take part in the MUDGIRL Run. It's outside my comfort zone, but life isn't comfortable, and I embrace that. This year is about my continued self-discovery and happiness. I may take some unplanned getaways and will take Samantha along for the ride. Melissa and I look forward to a September Sedona retreat—I can't wait! I will get an updated Akashic Record reading while I am there.

As I end this, I realize that the last four years, with their many ups and downs, are all part of me. I hope reading my book helps you see you can make it through sadness and darkness. Walk through the door into light and happiness. Pray when life is overwhelming, but also when life is good. Be thankful and find joy in small things. You can get through whatever challenges come your way by giving the problems to God and trusting through faith. Embrace your inner Divine Feminine or Divine Masculine and heal yourself.

Namaste!

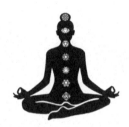

About The Author

V.C. grew up in a small Southern town. She lives with her son, Roman, and challenging dog, Crystal. V.C. runs a successful billing company. She enjoys walking and connecting with nature. Her favorite places are the beach and the mountains. V.C. loves to watch live music shows in small venues or outdoor amphitheaters. It's not unusual to find her at a metaphysical shop in search of a specific crystal or selecting a new tarot or oracle deck. Always looking for ways to enhance her spiritual growth, she attends retreats and participates in alternative healing modalities.

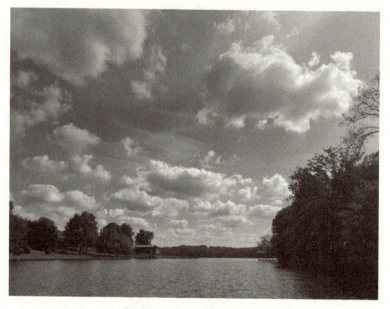

The lake where I find peace.

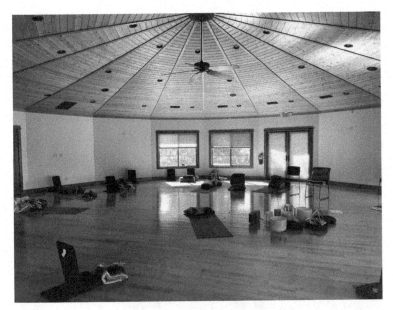

Mandala Hall at Elohee.

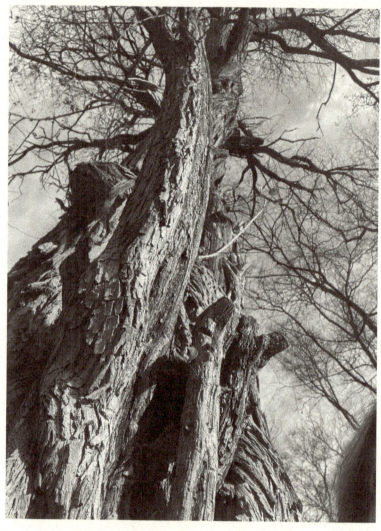

The tree where I ground at each morning.

Bibliography

BOOKS

Tolle, Eckhart. *The Power of Now: A Guide to Spiritual Enlightenment*. Vancouver, B.C. Namaste Publishing, 1999. Print.

The Power of Now: A Guide to Spiritual Enlightenment. Novato, California. New World Library, 2000. Audio.

SONGS

Clarence Carter, "Strokin," 1986, Single on *The Best of Clarence Carter*, Ichiban Records,
https://en.wikipedia.org/wiki/Clarence_Carter
Link Captured 5/09/22

Joe Cocker, "You Are So Beautiful," 1974, on *I Can Stand a Little Rain*, A&M Records.
https://en.wikipedia.org/wiki/You_Are_So_Beautiful
Link Captured 5/09/22

Commodores, "Just to Be Close to You," Single on *Hot on the Tracks*, Motown Records.
https://en.wikipedia.org/wiki/Just_to_Be_Close_to_You
Link Captured 5/09/22

Don Henley, "Heart of the Matter," 1990, Single on *The Heart of the Matter*, Geffen Records.
https://en.wikipedia.org/wiki/The_Heart_of_the_Matter_(song)
Link Captured 5/09/22

Jefferson Starship, "Miracles," 1975, Single on *Red Octopus*, Grunt/RCA Records.
https://en.wikipedia.org/wiki/Miracles_(Jefferson_Starship_song)
Link Captured 5/09/22

Kenny Rogers, "Love Will Turn You Around," 1982, Single on *Love Will Turn You Around*, Liberty Records.
https://en.wikipedia.org/wiki/Love_Will_Turn_You_Around
Link Captured 5/09/22

Seals and Crofts, "Diamond Girl," 1973, Single on *Diamond Girl* Soundtrack, Warner Bros. Records.
https://en.wikipedia.org/wiki/Diamond_Girl_(Seals_and_Crofts_song)
Link Captured 5/09/22

Sugarloaf, "Green-Eyed Lady," 1970, Single on *Sugarloaf*, Liberty Records.
https://en.wikipedia.org/wiki/Green-Eyed_Lady
Link Captured 5/17/22

The Stylistics, "You Make Me Feel Brand New," 1974, Single on *Rockin' Roll Baby* and *Let's Put It All Together*, Avco Records.
https://en.wikipedia.org/wiki/You_Make_Me_Feel_Brand_New
Link Captured 5/17/22

TV SHOWS

Little House on the Prairie, developed by Blanche Hanalis, Ed Friendly Productions and NBC Productions, 1974 – 1983.
https://en.wikipedia.org/wiki/Little_House_on_the_Prairie_(TV_series)
Link Captured 5/21/22

URLS

https://www.angelmessenger.net/the-ultimate-guide-to-angel-numbers-and-their-meanings/

https://www.ask-angels.com/spiritual-guidance/angels-and-numbers/#chapter7

https://www.ryanhart.org/angel-numbers/

http://geometricon.com/the-fibonacci-in-nature/

https://science.howstuffworks.com/math-concepts/fibonacci-nature.htm

https://en.wikipedia.org/wiki/Fibonacci_number

www.elohee.org

www.feliciagrant.com

VIDEOS

Amelia Caddy, Ph.D.
https://www.youtube.com/c/DrAmeliaCaddy/featured
Link Captured 5/17/22

Cristina "Black Rose"
Her channel is not currently active, but there's always a possibility of her return.
https://www.youtube.com/channel/UC9PMoSyKsMoSpVIHWfAClIw
Link Captured 5/24/22

Deb Spachman
https://www.youtube.com/c/DebDoesReadings
Link Captured 5/17/22

Eva Mozes Kor
https://youtu.be/gdgPAetNY5U
Link Captured 5/17/22

Sylvia Escalante
https://www.youtube.com/c/TheEnchantedWorldofTwinFlame
Link Captured 5/09/22